you can RENEW this item from
home by visiting our Website at
www.woodbridge.lioninc.org or by
calling (203) 389-3433

Food in the
Gilded Age

ROWMAN & LITTLEFIELD STUDIES IN FOOD AND GASTRONOMY
General Editor: Ken Albala, Professor of History,
University of the Pacific (kalbala@pacific.edu)
Rowman & Littlefield Executive Editor:
Suzanne Staszak-Silva (sstaszak-silva@rowman.com)

Food studies is a vibrant and thriving field encompassing not only cooking and eating habits but also issues such as health, sustainability, food safety, and animal rights. Scholars in disciplines as diverse as history, anthropology, sociology, literature, and the arts focus on food. The mission of **Rowman & Littlefield Studies in Food and Gastronomy** is to publish the best in food scholarship, harnessing the energy, ideas, and creativity of a wide array of food writers today. This broad line of food-related titles will range from food history, interdisciplinary food studies monographs, general interest series, and popular trade titles to textbooks for students and budding chefs, scholarly cookbooks, and reference works.

Food in the Gilded Age

What Ordinary Americans Ate

ROBERT DIRKS

ROWMAN & LITTLEFIELD
Lanham • Boulder • New York • London

Published by Rowman & Littlefield
A wholly owned subsidiary of The Rowman & Littlefield Publishing Group, Inc.
4501 Forbes Boulevard, Suite 200, Lanham, Maryland 20706
www.rowman.com

Unit A, Whitacre Mews, 26-34 Stannary Street, London SE11 4AB

British Library Cataloguing in Publication Information Available

Library of Congress Cataloging-in-Publication Data

Names: Dirks, Robert, 1942– author.
Title: Food in the Gilded Age : what ordinary Americans ate / Robert Dirks.
Description: Lanham : Rowman & Littlefield, [2016] | Series: Rowman &
  Littlefield studies in food and gastronomy | Includes bibliographical
  references and index.
Identifiers: LCCN 2015040482 | ISBN 9781442245136 (cloth : alk. paper)
Subjects: LCSH: Diet—United States—History—19th century. | Diet—United
  States—History—20th century. | Food habits—United States—History—19th
  century. | Food habits—United States—History—20th century.
Classification: LCC TX360.U6 D57 2016 | DDC 394.1/20973—dc23 LC record available
at http://lccn.loc.gov/2015040482

♾™ The paper used in this publication meets the minimum requirements of
American National Standard for Information Sciences—Permanence of Paper
for Printed Library Materials, ANSI/NISO Z39.48-1992.

Printed in the United States of America

Contents

Photographs

Tables

Recipes

Preface

Food consumption or dietary studies have been conducted in the United States for more than one hundred years. The very earliest, carried out by W. O. (Wilbur Olin) Atwater and his colleagues, embodied what was then cutting-edge science. Today that science has been surpassed. Interest in early dietaries these days has more to do with the history of nutrition than with the data the science produced.

That, however, is not the case here. This book revolves around the data. It rests on the conviction that carefully made observations never become outmoded even as the science that produced them develops different methods, novel theories, and new directions. The early accounts of food and eating habits that we find scattered among dusty and forgotten U.S. Department of Agriculture (USDA) bulletins are now of little use to nutritionists. But in the eyes of those curious about the food habits of a bygone era, they will forever represent valuable primary sources offering unusually fine-grained depictions of what Americans ate around the beginning of the twentieth century.

I became conscious of early dietaries and began to appreciate their value at the prompting of Nancy Duran, a librarian and part-time graduate student in history at Illinois State University. She introduced me to the extensive series of food inventories conducted prior to World War I under the auspices of the USDA's Office of Experiment Stations (OES). I read W. O. Atwater and Charles D. Wood's *Dietary Studies with Reference to the Food of the Negro in Alabama in 1895 and 1896* and came away impressed. Information about the eating habits of ordinary people who lived just four or five generations ago tend to be sketchy at best, but Atwater and Woods described the foods consumed back then in detail. Nancy and I collaborated on a couple of projects. We assembled an extensive bibliography of food consumption studies conducted in the United States prior to World War II.[1] We then used some of the data we located in order to write "African American Dietary Patterns at the Beginning of the 20th Century" for the *Journal of Nutrition*.[2] Donald McCormick, editor of the *Annual Review of Nutrition*, asked me to follow up with an article about the eating habits of other minorities. The idea for this book developed as I wrote that paper.[3]

The *Annual Review of Nutrition* serves a scientific community. I intend this book for readers interested in history. Nevertheless, I begin the same way I began my review article: by recounting the methods that Atwater and others used to produce their studies. Whether for purposes of science or to obtain historical understandings, we need to be mindful of how information was produced so that we can decide how much stock to put into it. The men and women who conducted the first dietaries were themselves very concerned about the quality of the information they produced. I refer to them as "early nutritionists" or "first-generation nutrition scientists," but in fact there was no science of nutrition at the time. Atwater and his collaborators were chemists. As such, they dedicated themselves to making careful and precise measurements. They took this commitment with them when they left their laboratories to observe food consumption in kitchens, dining rooms, and other mundane settings.

Surveying the results of early dietaries transports us to various parts of the United States during the Gilded Age. This name refers to an era of unprecedented disparity between rich and poor. The eating habits of both groups were, at the time, divided by region and ethnicity and catered to almost entirely by local producers and distributors.

Such was certainly the case in the recently annexed territory of New Mexico, the area I focus on in my introductory chapter. My particular concern here is the Mexican American kitchen, perhaps the most parochial of all American kitchens at the time. My introduction examines it from contrasting perspectives. On the one hand, it looks at the region and its food habits through the lens of ethnology. On the other hand, it relates the point of view of an Atwater-era dietary study. These examples help to distinguish between culinary history and nutrition history and assist in weighing their respective strengths and weaknesses. An account of the techniques and methods of early dietary studies closes out the chapter.

Chapter 2 takes us to southern Appalachia, where the text compares and contrasts the eating habits of backwoods farmers, townsfolk, and university students. Like the other chapters in this book, it reveals continuities with the past. In this instance, we see in cross-section a shift very much like that occurring today in parts of China and elsewhere in the developing world. This much-discussed nutrition transition involves a rejection of traditional diets composed mainly of vegetables in favor of diets containing far more animal products than in the past. This switch was under way in America's upland South at the end of the nineteenth century.

Chapter 3 attends to several African American communities and their eating habits. It examines dietary continuities and discontinuities across regional and class lines and looks at prototypical soul food diets in Alabama and Virginia several generations before the notion of soul food existed. The chapter explains how these local prototypes related to geography and commerce and why certain soul foods had little appeal to metropolitan blacks prior to the Great Migration.[4]

Chapter 4 concerns class differences and hunger. It describes the typical diet of well-to-do families from various parts of the East and Midwest and compares their eating habits with those of impoverished families in Chicago, New York City, Philadelphia, and Washington, DC. The chapter directs attention to the seasonality of late nineteenth- and early twentieth-century diets. It examines how the effects of seasonal changes varied by economic class and how annual hungers left their mark on members of the working class.

Chapter 5 inspects the food baskets of various immigrant groups. It compares the groceries they consumed, and it recounts the nutritional changes they experienced upon their arrival in the United States. Against a backdrop sketched by various European studies, these changes appear radical, particularly with respect to animal protein and animal fat consumption. The chapter ends by juxtaposing some of the nutritional changes experienced by the immigrants of yesteryear with those experienced by immigrants today.

Chapter 6 highlights institutional venues and work groups. It begins from the vantage point of college and university dining halls. These present reasonably standardized platforms from which to observe regional variations in the ways Americans eat. In addition, student dining facilities prove ideal for assessing the effects of gender on food consumption. Here the influences of strands of culture seemingly remote from the nutritional issues become apparent. There was no denying the culture-bound character of eating habits during the Gilded Age, even in seemingly rational and economically determined circumstances. Studies of three culturally disparate groups—elite college athletes, Chinese American field hands, and French Canadian lumberjacks—serve to illustrate this point.

A great many people deserve credit for helping me write this book. I am indebted to Deborah Dirks, Mike Doherty, Bob Hathway, Greg Koos, Bruce Kraig, Mike Matejka, Joan Mulcahy, Charley Schlenker, Joe Strano, and Janine Toth, all of whom took time to read and comment on chapters or pieces in the process of becoming chapters. I owe thanks, too, to Kathleen Christy, head of reference, Blount County Public Library; Dennis Daily, librarian for Archives and Special Collections at New Mexico State University; Eric Dulin, archivist at Cheyney University of Pennsylvania; Valerie E. Elliott, manager, Smith Library of Regional History, the Lane Libraries, Oxford, Ohio; and Micky Roberts, district director, Blount and Sevier County Tennessee Health Departments, for helping me track down images and information. Finally, I salute former students Tracy Abraham and Lawrence McBride, as well as my daughter, Kathryn Dirks, for their help entering page after page of nutrition data into my computer files. They certainly received ample exposure to one of the most tedious aspects of modern scholarship. Every time I called up a piece of information or ran an analysis of the data they transcribed, I had another occasion to appreciate their work.

1

Nutrition History

This book is about what Americans ate toward the end of the nineteenth century. Its last three decades, a period referred to as the "Gilded Age," were full of promise. Economic growth was brisk nearly everywhere, but instead of producing widespread prosperity, it mostly benefited those who were already rich and powerful. The standard of living among skilled wage earners increased, but the poor only became poorer thanks in large part to an enormous influx of unskilled labor from abroad. This amplified the disparities between the upper and lower classes and resulted in a number of serious social problems, including high levels of unemployment and drunkenness, broken families, child labor, violent street gangs, and overcrowded housing.

Abetted by popular support for programs that offered hope for a better society, a handful of scientists began making observations related to diet and nutrition. Their accounts of the kinds and the amounts of foods that ordinary people ate were unprecedented at the time. Today we have an abundance of experts dedicated to studying food consumption, but prior to the end of the nineteenth century, eating habits were, in effect, nobody's business. Eating was a matter too routine to give it much thought.

There were, of course, exceptions. History has bequeathed cookbooks and medical tracts telling us what previous generations were supposed to eat. Eyewitness historical accounts of meals have been recorded in diaries, memoirs, novels, traveler's accounts, and other sorts of literature. All of these represent useful sources of information; yet there are inevitably issues that diminish their value as windows on the past. Cookbooks and medical treatises, for instance, are essentially prescriptive. The big question about them always has to do with connections to the real world—to what extent did the written work affect or reflect popular practices? Purely descriptive accounts of yesteryear's eating habits raise concerns about selectivity. Narratives often tell of feasts and dishes consumed on special occasions. Authors usually have little or nothing to say about normal, everyday fare. Literary accounts, in general, are apt to address food haphazardly. On top of that, distinguishing the figurative from the literal can be difficult.

The prospect for a much more systematic and fine-grained historical picture brightened once food and its consumption became matters of scientific interest. European chemists started to collect information about the composition of foods and people's nutritional requirements in the early 1870s. W. O. Atwater, an American agricultural chemist who had been studying the composition of fertilizers, developed an intense interest in this work. He committed his laboratory at Wesleyan University to the analysis of foods. He visited Germany in order to study developments in the infant science of nutrition and wrote about how Americans could improve their lives by purchasing cheaper groceries. A series of articles written for the *Century Illustrated Monthly Magazine* and published in 1887 and 1888 brought Atwater's ideas to national attention.[1] Almost overnight, he became one of America's most famous scientists.[2]

Atwater's sudden rise to prominence owed a great deal to his no-nonsense attitude toward eating. His angle on food, which had little to do with enjoyment and nearly everything to do with economy, resonated well with a public convinced that the poor ate too extravagantly and that immigrants squandered their assets on victuals ill suited to American life.[3] Official recognition came close on the heels of his magazine series. To begin with, as soon as federal funds became available in 1887 to support an agricultural research station in each state, Atwater received an appointment as director of a new facility in Storrs, Connecticut. Soon afterward, the USDA invited him to Washington, DC, to take charge of the OES, which at this point needed someone to coordinate its expanding state programs.

Atwater undertook an ambitious series of studies while at the helm of the OES. He and his staff collected and analyzed foods from several areas of the United States. They sought to define people's nutritional needs through direct observation, and they worked to develop scientifically based recommendations for fulfilling those requirements at the lowest possible cost. To study nutritional needs and economical ways to meet them, Atwater authorized field studies in family households, boarding houses, college clubs, and other venues, most of which were meant to represent some particular segment of American society. These representations were ethnically and racially diverse, not so much because diversity had any scientific point but because Atwater understood the practical advantage of paying attention to immigrants and other minorities, whose numbers were growing rapidly and causing political headaches in Washington. Any program dedicated to learning about how such communities lived and promising to come up with ways to facilitate their assimilation was bound to find plenty of government support. As it turned out, this pragmatic approach to food and nutrition produced some terrific science having little or nothing to do with policy concerns.

RELATIONSHIP TO CULINARY HISTORY

W. O. Atwater died in 1907. The era defined by his research agenda continued for a few more years, but by the time the United States entered World War I, the science he founded was moving in new directions. Field research involving household and institutional food inventories became a method of the past, bringing an end to the list of products directly observed and weighed as a significant source of nutrition history.

Nutrition history, authored mainly by archaeologists, biological anthropologists, and economic historians, is not the same thing as food history.[4] The latter has attracted considerable attention over the past twenty years and consists of two principal branches. One of them is culinary history.[5] It covers food preparation, food service, tastes and styles, manners of eating, and how people used to think about foods. The goal of culinary history is to find meanings and develop understandings about the food habits of bygone eras. The other branch of food history, sociocultural studies, looks for relationships between food habits and other aspects of society.[6] Scholars undertaking sociocultural histories of foods are apt to look at matters in the context of economic and political patterns. Studies, for example, might aim to discover how newly introduced foods changed gender roles or patterns of trade. Or the purpose may be the other way around—for example, to show how family arrangements, industrial practices, or medical beliefs influenced food consumption. Nutrition history is not considered a third branch of food history, perhaps because, unlike the other two, it is starkly reductionistic. Nutrition history, for instance, pays more attention to grocery bags and food baskets than menus. It is about diet rather than cuisine. Dishes are of less concern than their ingredients and the nutrients they contain. The most salient matters about eating are frequencies and quantities. To some, these issues may sound prosaic, but there can be neither structure nor style without substance—in this instance, chemical substances essential to health. Consequently, nutrition history complements food history, tying it firmly to issues of human well-being.

MEXICAN AMERICAN DIETS IN THE RIO GRANDE VALLEY

Nutrition histories rely to a considerable extent on quantitative records. Food histories generally do not, mainly for want of opportunity. However, when quantification can be brought into play, it always sheds new light on the ways previous generations ate.

Two primary accounts of Mexican foods and eating habits in the Rio Grande Valley toward the end of the nineteenth century serve to illustrate how a few numbers can counterbalance rich narrative and deepen our understanding of the region's culinary history. The first, written by Colonel John Gregory Bourke of the U.S. Army, a great admirer of gastronome Jean Anthelme Brillat-Savarin, offers a firsthand survey of regional foods and food preparations. His narrative appears tailor-made for the future culinary historian.[7] The second account, prepared in two parts by Arthur Goss, professor of chemistry at the New Mexico College of Agriculture and Mechanical Arts, represents a small but substantial contribution to science, the kind of material on which, many years later, nutrition history thrives.[8]

Both authors possessed solid credentials, and both can be regarded as trustworthy. Goss served as vice-director of the New Mexico Agricultural Experiment Station from 1895 to 1900 and did extensive work on the composition of foods produced in the Las Cruces area. He analyzed, among other things, range beef, homemade lard, native white and blue corn, mesquite beans, and chili peppers. His interests beyond the laboratory embraced indigenous peoples and Mexican culture. Bourke, in addition to being a career soldier, was an ethnographer, ethnologist, linguist, and active member of the American Association for the Advancement of Science. While serving in Arizona, he took leave from his army unit in order to spend time among Indians, studying their customs.[9] His writings include two of the most peculiar works in the annals of anthropology: "The Urine Dance of the Zuni Indians of New Mexico" (published in 1885) and *Compilation of Notes and Memoranda Bearing upon the Use of Human Ordure and Human Urine* (which appeared in 1888).[10] Few nowadays know of these works (both of which were marked for restricted circulation), but, whatever their titles may suggest, Bourke intended them as serious ethnological contributions. Both sought to situate ritualistic and other uses of "vile aliment" within a broadly comparative framework. Bourke explained them as cultural scars etched by famine.

"The Folk Foods of the Rio Grande Valley and of Northern Mexico," published in the *Journal of American Folklore* in 1895, was a very different kind of work.[11] Devoid of any theoretical intensions, it offered a purely descriptive account of the traditional sustenance of the Mexican-American border region, which at that time was terra incognita as far as most of Bourke's compatriots were concerned. The paper, offered as the first comprehensive, English-language account of Mexican foods, traversed a wide range of topics. Beginning with capsule descriptions of forty-five indigenous vegetables and fruits used in regional cuisine, it wandered through Mexican cookery, telling of dozens of favorite dishes, some only sold by street vendors, some eaten exclusively during fiestas, and others served at home as family fare.

Goss's work, published as OES bulletins, appears exceedingly narrow by comparison. His observations, chronicled in 1895 and 1896, represented a total of eight weeks of fieldwork. He undertook his work during the months of April and May and all of it in the immediate vicinity of Las Cruces. Goss published just four dietaries collected from three Mexican American households. One of them, composed of a family located in Las Cruces proper, lived in "moderate circumstances." The other two families, both situated on a ranch outside of town, lived in extreme poverty.

Impoverished rural families usually clustered in small settlements. Some of them numbered as many as twenty households. Families generally settled along small streams and tilled the adjacent lands. In some instances, they owned the land; more often they rented. Living quarters generally consisted of thick-walled houses constructed of large, sun-dried adobe bricks. Among the poor, these dwellings normally contained no more than a single room with but one entrance and perhaps one or two windows protected by closely spaced wooden slats. Earthen floors and roofs constructed of brush covered with mud were customary. Sheep and other animal skins, used for sitting and sleeping, furnished the interiors. Water came from an outside well shared by neighbors.

Families living in town and in better circumstances adopted Anglo-American ways. Townspeople cooked on stoves and ate their meals seated on chairs at a table. The Las Cruces family studied by Goss owned an adobe brick house containing four rooms. Here meals included beef steaks, beef ribs, and hog's head. Goss's rural poor rarely ate meat products other than lard and tallow.

Cornmeal and wheat flour made up the bulk of everyone's diet. Among better-off families, wheat predominated over corn. The less fortunate ate mostly corn. Las Cruces folk favored a variety of blue corn with relatively soft

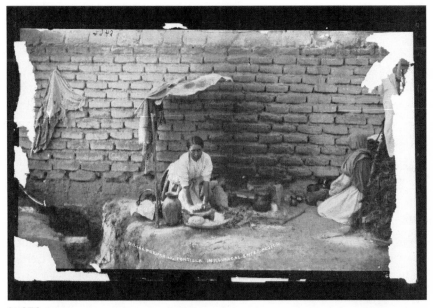

PHOTO 1.1
"Preparing Tortillas in Aguas Calientes, Mexico" (c. 1890). Woman mashing corn using *mano* and *matate*. (Photograph by William Henry Jackson. Courtesy of the Detroit Publishing Company Photograph Collection [LC-DIG-det-4a27118], U.S. Library of Congress, Prints and Photographs Division.)

kernels. It was crushed at home and used to make tortillas. The process began by boiling the kernels in water containing a little limestone. This softened the kernels, enabling removal of their skins, but some homemakers skipped this step and proceeded directly to grinding (see photo 1.1). This took place on a concave stone slab called a *metate*. There the kernels were crushed with a smaller, convex piece of stone, a *mano*, which was rubbed back and forth across the surface. This created a mush that was patted by hand into tortillas. Flour tortillas were flattened with a roller. The locally milled flour used to make them had a coarse texture and dark color. Both corn and flour tortillas were baked on a flat piece of iron greased with lard and suspended directly over the flames of an open fireplace.

In addition to wheat flour and corn, other common components of the local diet included beans, chilies, lard, eggs, potatoes, sugar, salt, and coffee. The beans, or *frijoles*, were boiled in small clay pots, usually along with a liberal measure of lard or "lard compound" (lard mixed with other fats and oils). In addition, a pot of *frijoles* almost always contained a substantial quantity of chilies. The chili was a common ingredient in many local dishes. Some called for powdered chilies, some for fleshy pieces, but in most instances preparations started with whole pods dried beforehand and in need of being stemmed and seeded. Once the stems and seeds were removed, the chilies could be pulverized with a *metate* or soaked in water preparatory to removing the skin. Once rehydrated, it took no more than a squeeze with the hand to jettison the skin.

Table 1.1 compares average daily nutritional intakes of Goss's impoverished rural subjects with those living in town. The table's format is more or less standard for the nutritional tables presented throughout this book.

Table 1.1.   Nutritional Values, Mexican American Diets, Las Cruces, Spring 1896–1897

HOUSEHOLDS	Animal CHO (g/m/d)	Animal Protein (g/m/d)	% Energy Animal Fat	% Energy Animal Products
Las Cruces	0	29	17	21
Rural Poor	0	1	13	14
HOUSEHOLDS	Vegetable CHO (g/m/d)	Total Protein (g/m/d)	Total Fat (g/m/d)	Total Energy (Cal/m/d)
Las Cruces	572	101	68	3305
Rural Poor	643	95	75	3657

RECIPE 1.1

NEW MEXICAN CHILE SALAD

The official spelling for the chili pepper native to New Mexico
(*Capsicum annuum*) is "chile."[1] New Mexicans savor them ripe
and red, but they prize them even more immature and green. The
green chile has come to be regarded as one of the cornerstones
of New Mexican cuisine. It can be enjoyed fresh roasted or dried
and powdered for use in the kitchen.

Alice Tipton, author of New Mexico's earliest cookbook, *New
Mexican Cookery*, urged her audience to be careful with chiles.[2]
She counseled readers never to use the skins and under no circumstances to eat the seeds. The skins have the toughness of
leather; the seeds, she warned, can burn a hole in your stomach.
This made it imperative for a chile to be blistered and seeded before cooking. Doing this properly required a blaze or a hot oven
and frequent turning. Once the skin of the chile puffed up, the pod
needed to be covered with a towel and allowed to steam. Then
the skin could be pulled away from the flesh, and an incision near
the stem allowed removal of the seeds.

A good way to enjoy the flavor of a New Mexican chile, minus any distractions introduced by other ingredients, is in chile
salad.[3] Take one or more dried green chiles or fresh ripe ones,
blister, and remove the skins and seeds. Soak the skinless pods
in saltwater overnight. In the morning, place the chiles in a pan
and pour just enough olive oil over them to cover the chiles. Then
heat the oil to almost boiling. Turn off the heat and allow to cool.
The chiles should remain in the oil for several hours before being taken out and served (save the remaining chile-infused oil for
salad dressings, sauces, etc.).

Tipton's recipe predates freezing. Outside of the harvest season, there was no alternative to dried chiles in her day. Nowadays, fresh chiles minus skins and seeds are available frozen
in specialty stores and from Internet shops at any time of the

year. Whole dried green chiles have become hard to find. Still, for those who want to prepare Tipton's salad using dried green chiles like native New Mexicans did in the past, the Chile Guy, an online supplier, sells four-ounce packages with the skins already removed from the pods.[4]

NOTES

1. "New Mexican Cuisine," *Wikipedia*, http://en.wikipedia.org/w/index.php?title=New_Mexican_cuisine&oldid=627481505.

2. Alice Stevens Tipton, *New Mexico Cookery* (Santa Fe: Bureau of Publicity of the State Land Office of the State of New Mexico, 1916), 11.

3. Ibid., 32.

4. The Chile Guy, http://www.thechileguy.com/.

The first numeric column tabulates average consumption of animal and vegetable carbohydrates. The next column shows protein intakes from animal sources and protein intakes from animal and vegetable sources combined. The following column reports the percent contribution of animal fat to total energy intake and average total fat consumption. In the absence of direct information, the extent to which animal fat contributes to total energy intake provides a good indication of the level of saturated fat in diets.[12] The final column represents the proportional energy contribution of animal products to diets and the average total intake of energy from animal as well as vegetable foods. Here the figures reveal that the diets of rural families were 86 percent vegetarian (14 percent of their energy came from animal sources).

Goss found the results of these dietaries, particularly the two compiled in 1895, astonishing. His data showed that one household took in absolutely no animal protein over the course of two weeks of observation. The other household consumed but 18 grams of egg protein over the course of 165 meals—

that is, less than 0.02 grams per day. Perhaps a mistake had been made or the situation at the time had been unusual.

Goss restudied one of the households the following year. This revealed the intake of some animal protein in the form of ten cents worth of beef ribs. Their nutritional value in terms of protein averaged out at approximately four grams per man per day, far less than reported for any other group in North America. By comparison, members of Goss's Las Cruces household took in around twenty-nine grams of protein per day. Another striking thing about the food lists that Goss collected was the small number of items they contain. Members of his middle-class household ate just seven and a half different foods per week. The households he monitored outside of town consumed only five distinct foods over the same period of time.

Foods not commonly consumed among the households totaled less than a dozen. Aliments occasionally noted among the rural poor included *fideos* (noodles usually used in soups), lentils, peas, onions, grape butter, and stick candy. In town, Goss saw rice, green onions, dried tomatoes, and apples.

On the subject of food variety, Colonel Bourke presented a remarkably different picture. For his portrait of a typical family, he created a "prudent little Mexican housewife" assisted by a servant girl. Bourke wrote of the latter being sent out to make purchases for a meal planned for later that day. The girl received instructions to buy onions, tomatoes, parsnips, pumpkin, and cabbage. Another day she might have been asked to get "juicy, sweet, scarlet *tunas* (prickly pears) . . . one or more each of *chirimoyas* (custard apples), bananas, figs, apples, oranges, grapes, mangoes . . . and a small slice of '*queso de tuna*.'"[13] Bourke's list of food consumed by his model family over the course of several days numbered fourteen items. Goss's systematic record for his relatively well-off Las Cruces family tallied just fifteen items *over a period of two weeks.* Judging by the presence of a servant, Bourke must have had in mind a family of above-average means. Goss professed that his Las Cruces family lived in moderate circumstances but that did not preclude owning a home with dirt floors. Here the only servant in the house was a seventeen-year-old daughter, and she did part-time work for another family.

Bourke had no interest in being as specific as Goss. The colonel preferred the ethnographic present, a literary device that compresses observations made over a long period into an ubiquitous here and now. This permitted him to make foods actually served over a period of several days or weeks part of an idealized account of a single day. The idea that he was creating a false impression of variety probably never arose. After all, Bourke's survey, with its long list of foods encountered over years of travel across great expanses, was about variety. As a literary device, a household with a servant created a better opportunity to write about the region's cuisine than an impoverished family eating tortillas and *frijoles* day after day. This explains why the Mexican "rustic," the term Bourke applied to peasants, appeared as no more than a footnote in his culinary survey.

METHOD AND TECHNIQUES IN EARLY DIETARIES

There is no question that Goss's report on Mexican food habits was more exact than Bourke's, but to what extent was Goss's account representative? There is no telling. Scientific sampling had yet to be worked out. Scientists selected subjects thought to be typical of one or another area or community. To lend credibility to their selections, Atwater and his colleagues solicited expert opinions and relied on well-informed collaborators to identify and help recruit subjects.

The preferred protocol for conducting dietary research called for a fieldworker to visit his or her subjects at least once a day, at which time every food item acquired since the fieldworker's last visit was to be registered and weighed. This made fieldwork tedious and time consuming for everyone concerned. H. B. Frissell's study of African American families in Virginia's Great Dismal Swamp, for instance, entailed a fifteen-mile round trip by horse and wagon every day.[14] Along the way, foods intended for the table had to be logged and placed on a scale in as many as a dozen different households. Kitchen refuse and table wastes, normally fed to the chickens and pigs, were collected at each stop and weighed as well. A pail of animal feed left behind compensated families for saving their garbage until the next day's weighing.

Researchers tried alternatives to daily house calls. Ellen Richards and Amelia Shapleigh experimented in Philadelphia in 1892 with questionnaires and self-kept account books.[15] However, the next year, when they recruited members of Chicago's Hull House women's club for a project that relied almost entirely on self-reporting, their study yielded suspiciously high nutritional values for households that were supposed to be very poor. Atwater and A. P. Bryant tried self-reporting again three years later, once more in Chicago. Their subjects consisted of better-off families and relatively assimilated immigrants;

however, the results did nothing but erode confidence in self-reporting. Records kept by research subjects consistently declared food intakes greater than those based on twice-daily visits by professional staff.[16]

Researchers also had to contend with suspicions and hostile attitudes. Charles Wait, a chemistry professor at the University of Tennessee, ran into trouble in Tennessee's Chilhowee Mountains because, as he put it, few householders seemed "disposed to let their bills of fare or their cost of living be known."[17] Wait wisely sought help from a colleague, A. F. Gilman, a native of the area. Gilman knew the local culture, and instead of trying to explain the project to people as a scientific exercise, he obtained cooperation by proposing some elementary reciprocity. In exchange for a small but much-appreciated sum of cash, family members obliged themselves to be more forthcoming and tolerant of daily inquiries. Less easily overcome were the political mistrusts that existed in cities like Chicago and Pittsburgh, where rumors circulated that investigators wanted to see how cheaply people could eat so that employers could cut wages accordingly. Families in these circumstances came under pressure from their neighbors not to participate in dietary studies.[18]

Researchers sought to engender trust by working through well-regarded local agencies. Working in Philadelphia, Ellen Richards, based at the Massachusetts Institute of Technology's chemistry department, entered into a cooperative relationship with the College Settlement Association.[19] Atwater and his associates followed her example in Chicago, New York City, and Pittsburgh.[20] Tuskegee and Hampton Institutes lent their good names to studies of African American food habits.[21] In addition, institute and agency staff members did much of the fieldwork. Atwater and Woods, for instance, had J. W. Hoffman of the Tuskegee Institute to thank for a robust set of dietaries gathered from local African American farmers and field hands.[22] Isabelle Delaney, a physician dedicated to work among the poor, used her deep understanding of tenement life to unlock doors on New York's Lower East Side, where she compiled most of the fifty-nine dietaries published by the OES.[23]

By whatever means, the idea was to keep an accurate running inventory of food supply. For a household, this entailed listing and weighing all of the provisions on hand at the beginning of the study, and from that point on keeping a tally of every food entering the premises. The itemizing and weighing continued for at least a week and occasionally went on for as long as a month. The enumerations concluded with some calculations. The quantities of food on hand at the start of the inquiry and those registered over the succeeding days were totaled. Wastes and foods still on the shelf at the end of the study were deducted from the total. The remainder represented net household consumption.

Net household consumption, because households differ in size and composition, was not a useful statistic for comparative purposes. To create a more serviceable number, investigators reduced net consumption to adult male equivalents or "man-units."[24] They accomplished this by establishing a moderately active male of average weight (150 lb. or 68 kg) as a hypothetical standard against which others' nutritional needs were measured. Studies showed, for example, that a male weighing 150 pounds and engaged in strenuous activity needed about 20 percent more food than the standard, moderately active male. Thus, a man at hard labor counted as 1.2 man-units. A moderately active woman generally consumed about 80 percent of the standard and, therefore, equaled 0.8 man-units. The adult male equivalent of a fourteen- to sixteen-year-old boy also came to 0.8 man-units. A girl between fourteen and sixteen amounted to the nutritional equivalent of 0.7 man-units, and so it continued down to babies less than two years old (the nutritional equivalent of 0.3 man-units). To represent consumption in terms of man-units, researchers multiplied the number of meals consumed by each person within a particular household by their adult male equivalent. They then divided the net household consumption by the sum of the products to arrive at consumption per man-unit. Finally, because dietaries were conducted over various lengths of time, investigators divided consumption per man-unit by three (the standard number of daily meals) to produce per-day values.[25] For substances such as protein or fat, consumption was typically expressed as grams per man per day (g/m/d). Energy intake was typically stated in terms of kilocalories per man per day (represented here as Cal/m/d).

Procedures in the laboratories were relatively straightforward. Chemists analyzed samples of foods "as purchased" and in a relatively unprocessed state. The results were used to assign nutritional values to similar items listed in the accompanying household inventories. Nutrients around 1900 consisted exclusively of protein, fat, and carbohydrates.[26] For every food logged in a dietary, researchers tabulated weight, energy value, and purchase cost. Costs for homegrown foods were equated to prices at the nearest market.

The undeveloped state of nutritional knowledge at the time makes it tempting to render early studies somewhat more meaningful by using current nutrition tables to extrapolate presumptive values from the published data. The sticking point is that the nutritional contents of fruits and vegetables have changed significantly over the years. One study comparing twenty fruits and twenty vegetables grown in the 1930s and the 1980s showed marked reductions in mineral contents.[27] These included statistically significant reductions in magnesium, iron, copper, and potassium in the fruits and calcium, magnesium, copper, and sodium in the vegetables. Besides that, the water content had increased significantly in the fruits, with a corresponding and significant decrease in dry matter. These changes could be due to measurement problems, historical differences in the varieties raised, altered growing conditions, or a combination of these and other factors. No one knows for sure. Uncertainty also prevails with respect to vitamins. In a nutshell, there exist no bases to presume beyond historical values.

Fortunately, it is possible to work around the missing nutrient issue using the detailed food lists found in the published dietaries of the period. These lists constitute a rough-and-ready measure of dietary variety. This book uses the number of different foods consumed over specified periods as a measure of dietary variety. Thinking about diets in terms of foods and the variety of foods in a person's diet lacks the specificity of citing mineral and vitamin intakes, but it subsumes greater complexity. It allows that food contains a myriad of biologically active components and that intake is not completely described by the limited set of nutrients conventionally referred to in the journals. Attention to variety recognizes the importance of balanced nutrition and captures a dimension of diet positively associated with good health.[28]

The way dietaries appeared in print remained standard throughout the Atwater era. Most studies of individual households and other groups were numbered in order of publication. Many were published in sets, often with a regional or topical theme—for example, OES Bulletin 31, *Dietary Studies at the University of Missouri in 1895, and Data Relating to Bread and Meat Consumption in Missouri* (1896), or OES Bulletin 221, *Dietary Studies in Rural Regions in Vermont, Tennessee, and Georgia* (1909).[29]

Whether published alone or as part of a set, a dietary always contained one or more tables listing the foods consumed and their nutritional contents. Instead of using broad categories such as "meat" or "beef," authors specifically indicated "porterhouse steak," "rump roast," "shoulder clod," and so forth.

Families typically did not eat greens in dietaries; they specifically ate lettuce, turnip greens, or watercress.

For households, each dietary within a collection usually contained a list of members and some more or less pertinent remarks followed by tables reporting collective food use and nutrition. Dietary no. 44, titled "Dietary of a Tinner's Family in Indiana," was typical. It appeared under the authorship of Winthrop Stone in OES Bulletin 32, *Dietary Studies at Purdue University, Lafayette, Ind., in 1895* (1896).[30] In it, Stone states that work began April 22 and continued for ten days. He lists as household members a fifty-five-year-old man, a twenty-year-old man, and a forty-eight-year-old woman. He said nothing about their relationship to one another (early dietaries usually did not), but he noted that over the course of his investigation, together they consumed 103 meals with 2 additional meals served to visitors. Stone wrote that everyone in the household was healthy and quite active, but they were not hearty eaters. He went on to relate that the men owned a small business and worked less hours than hired laborers. He noted the men smoked moderately, but they were not otherwise addicted to stimulants or narcotics. Not included in Stone's narrative but often recorded in dietaries were income, type of housing, cost of rent, and observations about sanitary conditions. In addition, published studies occasionally reported their subjects' weights. Some reports described distinctive food habits. Only in rare instances did authors write about other cultural practices or portray social environments.

First-generation nutritionists altogether published more than five hundred dietaries between 1885 and 1916. These, together with a handful of budget studies (budgetaries) put together by various agencies, provide data about food consumption in nearly 350 households, a few of them the subject of two or more inquiries conducted at different times of the year. Scientists of the era also produced statistics on food consumption for more than forty individuals, seventeen groups of college students, thirteen work groups and sports teams, eleven boarding houses, and a handful of public and private care institutions, including hospitals, nurseries, and orphanages.

These numbers are miniscule compared to those rung up in modern nutrition surveys. However, comparing a series of carefully conducted food inventories to today's studies based on recall questionnaires or food diaries is not unlike comparing a handmade product to one that is mass-produced. Administering recall questionnaires and food diaries is a lot cheaper than actually counting and weighing groceries. Questionnaires distributed to as many people as feasible became necessary once researchers began to count micronutrients, and they found that vitamin and mineral intakes tended to be far more variable than the consumption of macronutrients. Big samples reduced the risk of error. This is an especially important consideration when health and well-being are at stake. However, big samples are not so salient to the study of history, especially in a field where an excerpt from a book of travels or an entry in a diary can be taken as evidence of a general pattern. By the standards of food history, even three or four systematically collected food records, such as the Mexican American dietaries published by Goss, can represent a significant contribution to knowledge.

STRUCTURE OF A DIET

Historians and social scientists involved in food studies complement the perspective of nutrition scientists by describing cultural understandings and social practices that affect food consumption. Nancy Duran and I brought an anthropological perspective to our historical study of African American food consumption by developing a cultural model to interpret dietary data.[31] The work of John Bennett, Harvey Smith, and Herbert Passin inspired our model.[32]

Many years ago, Bennett, Smith, and Passin developed a kind of structural representation of diet in order to help understand dietary changes in southern Illinois in the late 1930s. Their model envisioned a typical diet as having three parts: a primary core, a secondary core, and a periphery. The primary core consisted of staples and other basics, as well as "traditional foods" (survivals from earlier dietary patterns). Secondary core foods encompassed more recent introductions, items gaining popularity because of modernization and expanding markets. The peripheral diet consisted of novel products and luxury foods. These appeared on the family table only on rare occasions.

Duran and I quantified Bennett, Smith, and Passin's model. We made the primary core the most frequently used foods in a community, setting the threshold at 50 percent. In other words, we designated as primary foods those that were found in at least half of the households in a community.[33] Foods in the secondary core failed to qualify as primary, but they appear in at least a quarter of the inventories recorded. Peripheral items are those noted less often. The underlying assumption is that the frequency with which a food is served has more pertinence culturally than the quantity consumed. A meat-

and-potatoes culture is one in which people eat meat and potatoes every day. More or less meat and more or less potatoes are primarily matters of economic wherewithal, not matters of cultural practice or understanding.

Of course, cultural matters are always relative, and when it comes to food, much depends on the time of year. Core items in season (zucchini in late summer) become peripheral out of season (e.g., in February). We need not automatically regard traditional foods as core items, but certainly turkey might be a core item in many American family diets around the Thanksgiving holiday. Afterward, it generally fades to the periphery of the typical diet and certainly by midyear may be regarded as culturally out of place as a family dinner item.

2

Mountaineers and a Nutrition Transition in Appalachia

In recent years, the developing world has experienced sharp increases in obesity, hypertension, diabetes, and mortality due to cardiovascular diseases.[1] The causes include increasingly sedentary lifestyles and some fundamental changes in diet. Chinese consumers, for example, have shifted toward foods with higher energy densities. They have increased their consumption of foods from animal sources, and they now eat considerably more fat than they did just a couple of decades ago. These changes, which are indicative of a major nutrition transition, have occurred elsewhere in the world.[2] Some parts of the industrialized West experienced them more than two centuries ago. They were afoot in southern Appalachia toward the end of the Gilded Age.

The coincidental creation of a large and varied collection of early dietaries captured southern Appalachia's nutrition transition in progress. Charles Wait, a chemistry professor at the University of Tennessee, initiated this fortunate accident in 1895, when he began studying students' eating habits.[3] A newspaper article brought his research to public attention and prompted several Knoxville families to invite him to evaluate their diets. Soon afterward, Wait turned his attention some twenty miles south of Knoxville and began inquiries at Crooked Creek, a remote community of Mountaineers.[4] His work expanded into nearby Maryville, a then burgeoning factory town. Inventories representing food use for no less than sixty-three households resulted from these efforts. About the same time, H. C. White, a chemist at the University of

Georgia, was doing similar work.[5] He, too, began working with students, but soon he widened his investigations to include Habersham, Rabun, and White counties in the mountainous northeastern corner of the state.

CROOKED CREEK

Wait began his work in East Tennessee for both practical and romantic reasons. On the practical side, he was W. O. Atwater's man, a government scientist committed to learning about local eating habits and applying whatever knowledge he might gain to public education and social betterment. The Mountaineer's diet had a reputation for being simple and inexpensive. It may not have been perfectly complete or well balanced, but as far as anyone knew, it caused no harm. Wait entertained the common notion that life in the mountains remained faithful to a less complicated and healthier past. Studying Mountaineers provided a glimpse of long-gone but better days. Mountain folks, as Wait pictured them, descended from the pioneers who first crossed the Appalachians. As valley towns in the Tennessee River system became increasingly civilized, those "wild, lawless characters" who did not move west retreated into the mountains, where their descendants remained "almost as primitive and isolated as their pioneer ancestors."[6]

Crooked Creek, located in the sparsely populated Chilhowee Mountains, certainly had a primitive look. Households lay scattered along the creek for several miles, and residents lived in rudimentary cabins. Built from logs with a brick or stone chimney running up an outside wall, their design had remained unchanged for at least a century. An ordinary dwelling consisted of two rooms—one for sleeping, the other for cooking and eating. Sometimes these were windowless; more often they had a shuttered opening in the wall, unframed and without glass. Rooms contained but a few furnishings, perhaps some beds, a table, and a few rough chairs. Mountaineers normally had no use for embellishments like wallpaper, curtains, and carpets. The household inventory of a Civil War veteran and his wife listed three beds, ten chairs, three tables, a cook stove, a "safe" for dishes, another for food (to protect it from vermin), and a clock.[7] Owning a cooking stove was unusual. Most homemakers prepared meals over the fireplace.

Families typically farmed. Crooked Creek's farms varied in size from small lots to cultivations of seventy-five acres (about thirty hectares) or more.

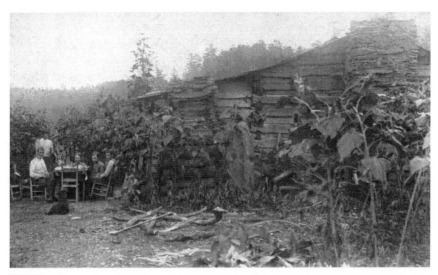

PHOTO 2.1
"A. J. Dorsey's Cabin. Family at Breakfast" (1886). The Mountaineers of East Tennessee scratched a meager living from their ridge-and-valley lands in the midst of America's Gilded Age. (Photograph by William Cox Cochran. Courtesy of the William Cox Cochran Great Smoky Mountains Photographic Collection [wcc047], Special Collections Library, University of Tennessee.)

Many families, some of them extended by the inclusion of married offspring, worked small, difficult pieces of land, often rented, in exchange for a portion of the crop. Farmers raised corn, wheat, beans, potatoes, sweet potatoes, and clover. Some families had gardens producing vegetables for home use. Almost everyone relied on their own corn, which they carried to the local mill for grinding. Their livestock included cows, ducks, hogs, horses, and mules, though not every household in the community kept animals.

Crooked Creek stood well off the beaten path. A few men worked for wages at a nearby sawmill, some at the local gristmill, but otherwise little cash changed hands. Residents traded for the things they could not provide for themselves. Provisions like salt and sugar could be had locally, but obtaining less common items required hitching up the mules and taking the day to go to Maryville, a journey of eight miles over very rough roads.

Table 2.1 shows the late summer fare of a typical Crooked Creek household observed over the course of fourteen days. It includes peripheral foods

Table 2.1. Typical Diet at Crooked Creek, Late Summer 1904

	Meat and Dairy	Grains and Dried Legumes	Fats, Oils, Sugars, and Starches	Roots and Tubers	Other Vegetables	Fruits and Misc.
Primary Core	salt pork	cornmeal wheat flour	lard			
Secondary Core	skimmed milk buttermilk		butter brown sugar	potato		
Periphery		dried bean	sugar molasses	sweet potato onion	cabbage	

inventoried in as few as 10 percent of the households studied, but even so it contains just fifteen commodities, fewer victuals than were inventoried in Goss's Mexican American dietaries. An exhaustive list—a catalog of every foodstuff seen in the community—includes only five more items: apple jelly, butter beans, green corn, sauerkraut, and string beans. By Wait's calculation, the primary core of the diet (cornmeal, wheat flour, lard, and salt pork) made up three-fourths of what household members actually ate. The secondary core included three dairy products (skimmed milk, buttermilk, and butter), and from there on everything else came from vegetable sources. Yet, aside from grains, families did not often eat vegetables other than potatoes. What is more, fruits of any kind were extremely rare, even though fieldwork took place in August and September, two very productive months for the gardens and orchards in nearby Maryville.

FRONTIER FOOD HABITS

The dearth of fruits and vegetables in Crooked Creek ought to have come as no surprise to Wait, especially given his view that Mountaineers remained true to the ways of the pioneers. Travelers along the southern frontier a century or so earlier had complained repeatedly about the absence of fruits and vegetables.[8] Fried pork, cornmeal, and coffee made up the early settlers' mainstays from the eastern Highlands all the way to the Rockies.[9] The wheat flour in Mountaineer dietaries was a relative newcomer to southern Appalachia, and people used it much as cornmeal had been used for generations.[10] Because corn could not be baked into loaves, neither would wheat—hence biscuits rather than loaves of bread.

Corn preceded wheat throughout the South because it yielded more return for less effort.[11] Compared to wheat, corn bore four times as much grain per acre, and it was ready to eat "green" in about six weeks. On top of that, early settlers did not have to spend time on careful field preparation, and they could let a mature crop stand in the field during the winter, harvesting ears as needed.

Corn was no great trouble to put on the table, either. It was boiled or roasted fresh and eaten off the cob or cut off the cob and fried. Left to dry, it was ground into meal and made into a variety of breads or cakes. The simplest consisted of just meal and water, perhaps with some salt. Homemakers added baking soda, milk, buttermilk, lard, or eggs as enrichments. The batter went into a Dutch oven that had been greased with a piece of pork rind and dusted with bit of cornmeal to prevent the bread from sticking. The oven was then preheated in the fireplace. Once hot, it was filled with batter, returned to the fireplace, and buried in hot coals. It normally took about twenty minutes to bake bread this way.[12] Cornmeal was also made into mush and griddle cakes.

Hominy required whole kernels of dried corn. To make it, a homemaker soaked or boiled the kernels in water containing a lime or wood ash. This removed the skins.[13] The kernels then might be sun dried and cooked whole. More often, they were ground and boiled and served as hominy grits, a popular breakfast dish.[14]

The unmodified term *grits* usually referred to coarsely ground cornmeal. Some folks applied the word to meal that would not go through a sifter. These bits were washed, added with some salt to a pot of boiling water, and simmered. They cooked to the consistency of oatmeal and were ready to eat in about thirty minutes.[15]

Pork became a southern staple after the frontier gave way to settlements and wild game became scarce. Again, species characteristics determined the matter.[16] No other domestic animal prospered as well as pigs did and with so little husbandry. A pig born in the spring required no pasture and put on weight far more rapidly than cattle or sheep. As it rooted through the remaining forest or scavenged fields, it converted plant materials to meat approximately seven times more efficiently than the competing ruminants.

The pig became a part of almost everything on the southern table. Lard, rendered from pig fat, went into cornbreads as shortening. Cracklings—the bits of crisp flesh left over from lard making—were mixed with cornmeal batter and baked into bread. Lard ranked as one of the two chief mediums of cooking. The other was water, which is to say that most dishes were either fried or boiled. Potatoes might be fried. Vegetables such as cabbage, turnip greens, and collards were apt to be boiled, but not without adding some salt pork for extra flavor. Settlers cured pork by packing parts of the pig in a box covered with salt for a month or more and then slowly smoking them. Meat processed in this way kept for many months.

Emily Stevens Maclachlan's 1932 study of the southern diet and its history led her to conclude the most striking thing about it was its "extreme cheapness."[17] Corn and pork fat plus plenty of sugar and molasses made for low-cost concentrated energy, while frying and boiling were the quickest, easiest means of cooking. Maclachlan speculated that these cheap and easy ways resulted from the necessities of work and time pressures on women.[18] It did not take long to fry a little fat and corn pone before mealtime. The vegetables could be left boiling from the time a housewife left her fireplace after breakfast until she arrived home again that evening. Even for people not working in fields, there was enough exhausting labor to leave them looking for the quickest and easiest means of cooking. It thus came as no accident that early settlers developed a studied disinterest in food. Meals were a matter of dispatch, and a manner of hurried eating became the cultural standard.

That all of this persisted in Appalachia did not come about, as Wait imagined, because the advance of civilization chased wild, lawless characters into the hills. Rather, it continued because developers on the lookout for investment opportunities found nothing in the hills that grabbed their attention. Capital, in effect, moved west, leaving behind what Horace Kephart called a "Land of Do Without," a materially impoverished region without the physical and social infrastructure needed for further development.[19] Like the piney woods of Alabama and Mississippi about the middle of the nineteenth century and the Big Thicket of East Texas a decade or more into the twentieth century, southern Appalachia and places like Crooked Creek retained the character of a newly settled area long after the frontier moved westward.

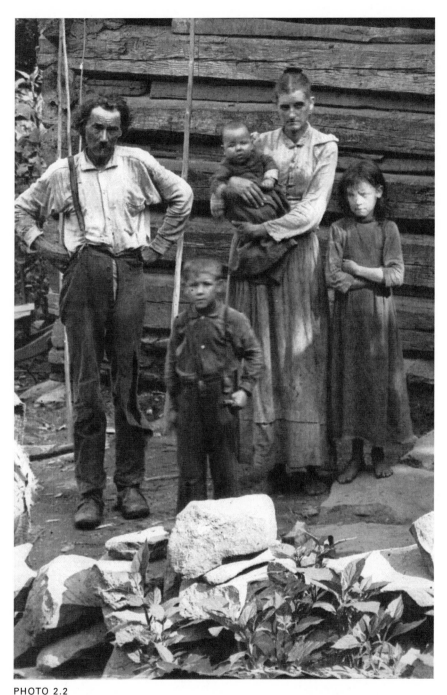

PHOTO 2.2

"Mountain Family" (no date). Residents of Tennessee's Blount County, citizens of the Land of Do Without. (Photograph by William Orland Garner. Courtesy of the W. O. Garner Digital Photograph Collection [bcapp00145], University of Tennessee Libraries/ Blount County Public Library, Maryville, TN.)

NORTHEAST GEORGIA

H. C. White's data for northeastern Georgia, collected in 1902, represent the eating habits of eleven Mountaineer households situated well within the borders of the Land of Do Without.[20] White recruited a local, a physician named De Buboeay, to conduct his inventories. De Buboeay's practice, located in the town of Tallulah Falls, the Saratoga Springs of the South, thrived on tourists. During the summer, five trains a day brought hundreds of them to marvel at the falls and the beauty of Tallulah Gorge.

Tallulah Falls boasted seventeen hotels connected by wooden streets, but just outside of town folks lived much as they did around Crooked Creek, some one hundred miles to the northwest. Men built log cabins for their families and occupied themselves with farmwork. For the most part, they raised corn, potatoes, and apples. Occasionally they cut wood and collected bark for area tanneries. Women looked after the children, kept house, cultivated kitchen gardens, cooked, and helped in the fields. Meals usually consisted of bacon, milled corn, vegetables, and dried apples, all produced locally. Families traded for flour and sugar at the country store.

Apples constituted important items of trade and had immense importance in the local diet. This derived from their potential for keeping throughout the winter and providing nourishment as other foods became scarce. Storage was especially easy in the mountains, where the fruit ripened late and the temperatures were cold enough for the harvest to remain in good condition for months. In the Tallulah Falls area, the Rabun Bald (or Rabun Ball), a now extinct variety of apple native to Rabun County, was held in especially high esteem because it did not ripen until November and could be kept barreled or boxed in a cold room until March.[21] As an alternative to storing fresh apples, farmers sometimes dried them in the sun or a heated "dry house." They also preserved them by bleaching or smoking, a process that involved exposing slices to sulfur fumes in a covered barrel. The treated slices were stored in a crock or box through the winter and used to make fried apples, apple fritters, and many other apple dishes native to southern cookery.

The centrality of apples among Georgia's Mountaineers differentiated their diet from that of Tennessee's, but otherwise folks ate pork, lard, cornmeal, and wheat—the same primary commodities listed in table 2.1 for Crooked Creek. De Buboeay also found whole milk and cowpeas (black-eyed peas) in

APPLE COBBLER

This recipe comes from *The Foxfire Book of Appalachian Cookery*, a book about the kitchen culture of northeastern Georgia that essentially revisits the area explored nutritionally by H. C. White and his assistant De Buboeay.[1] Foxfire books are the offspring of the Foxfire Program and its *Foxfire Magazine*. The program originated as the brainchild of high school English teacher Eliot Wigginton, who envisioned it as a class project. The idea was for his students at the Rabun Gap–Nacoochee School to interview their relatives about traditions and local ways of life. Wigginton and his students began writing up their interviews as magazine articles in 1966. These articles detailed numerous aspects of mountain culture and its history. Foxfire launched a series of books, each devoted to particular facets of mountain life, in 1972.

The Foxfire Book of Appalachian Cookery contains several recipes for cobbler, a kind of deep-dish pie minus the bottom crust. Ruth Cabe, one of the many informants who contributed her knowledge to Foxfire, referred to it as the region's "usual pie."[2] A cobbler might feature blackberries, rhubarb, cherries, or whatever. In the case of apple cobbler, fresh slices of the fruit were used when it was in season; dried slices were used in the winter. Dorothy Beck, another of Foxfire's contributors, made her apple cobbler using five or six apples cut into cubes.[3] These she placed in a sheet cake pan, pouring a little water over them. Next she added a topping, using a cup of sugar, a cup of flour, and a half cup of butter. Dorothy mixed these ingredients thoroughly. She then sprinkled the mixture over the top of her cubed apples. The pan went into the oven to bake at 350 degrees Fahrenheit for twenty or thirty minutes or until done. This cobbler was sufficient for ten to fifteen servings.

NOTES

1. Linda Garland Page and Eliot Wigginton, eds., *The Foxfire Book of Appalachian Cookery* (New York: Gramercy Books, 1984).

2. Ibid., 222.

3. Ibid., 223.

more than 50 percent of the households he studied, but these items appeared
exclusively in autumn and winter inventories.

BACKWOODS NUTRITION

Table 2.2 displays the average nutritional contents of diets in Crooked Creek,
northeastern Georgia, and Maryville. It also represents nutrition among semi-
skilled laborers in two southern towns and students at two southern universities. The values for northeastern Georgia are broken down into two categories,

Table 2.2.   Average Nutritional Values, Various Diets, Georgia and Tennessee, 1895–1904

PEOPLE & PLACES	Animal CHO (g/m/d)	Animal Protein (g/m/d)	% Energy Animal Fat	% Energy Animal Products	% Budget Animal Products	
Students (fall and winter)	15	57	35	42	52	
Mechanics (fall and winter)	12	56	45	52	64	
Maryville (winter)	16	26	27	32	47	
Northeast Georgia* (winter)	4	9	23	24	40	
Northeast Georgia (late summer and fall)	1	11	21	21	33	
Crooked Creek (late summer)	11	16	27	30	47	
PEOPLE & PLACES	Vegetable CHO (g/m/d)	Total Protein (g/m/d)	Total Fat (g/m/d)	Total Energy (Cal/m/d)	Variety (foods/week) Avg	Variety (foods/week) Max
Students (fall and winter)	479	106	151	3536	21	57
Mechanics (fall and winter)	842	114	207	3865	12	14
Maryville (winter)	549	88	128	3662	7	13
Northeast Georgia (winter)	676	84	118	3557	6	7
Northeast Georgia (late summer and fall)	944	117	159	5669	5	7
Crooked Creek (late summer)	540	82	132	3726	3	6

* Values for northeast Georgia exclude families of landowners.

one pertaining to late summer and fall (dietaries collected in September and early November) and the other specific to winter.

Notice that table 2.2 contains a column of data not represented in our previous tabulation of nutritional values (table 1.2). The upper level of the final column reports the average proportion of household food budgets spent on foods from animal sources. The lower tier, divided into subcolumns, represents dietary variety assessed in two different ways. The first, which refers to average variety, stands for the mean number of foods used per week of observation. The second, maximum variety, shows the greatest number of foods consumed by any one household (or group of students) during that particular study. This measure is less sensitive than the first due to disparities in the duration of inventories among the various sets of subjects being compared.

The table exposes some remarkable similarities and differences. One obvious correspondence between Tallulah Falls and Crooked Creek was the monotony of the diets. In neither place did the most varied diet exceed seven different foods per week. Toward the end of the growing season, when a multitude of fruits and vegetables ought to have been available, dietary variety in both Crooked Creek and the Tallulah Falls area was considerably less than what was computed for the town of Maryville in the dead of winter. In addition, the intake of animal protein proved to be exceedingly low in both backwoods locations. The average winter intake in northeastern Georgia was little more than one-third of the winter average for Maryville. Diets low in protein and containing excessive fat appear to have produced unhappy consequences in Crooked Creek, where Wait discovered significantly overweight or obese children in five households (26 percent of the total number) and an underweight child in another.[22]

The most remarkable nutritional differences between Crooked Creek and northeastern Georgia related to the huge discrepancy in energy intakes for late summer and early autumn. Georgia's highlanders at that time of year took in well over 5,000 Cal/m/d, on average over 2,000 Cal/m/d more than the residents of Crooked Creek. Much of this energy came from vegetable sources, including apples. Did the people around Tallulah Falls require much more energy than the folks along Crooked Creek? There is no way to answer that question conclusively. However, what with the higher elevation and colder temperatures and employment in the woodcutting industry, it would seem very likely that such was the case.[23]

Whatever the causes, it is noteworthy that the difference in energy intake between Tallulah Falls and Crooked Creek was seasonal, and by winter the average energy content of diets in northeastern Georgia was about 60 percent of what it had been two or three months earlier (see table 2.2). A running average beginning in September at 4,959 Cal/m/d tops out in November at a whopping 6,142 Cal/m/d, and then it plummets in January and February to 3,557 Cal/m/d. There was considerable variation among households during the winter, and some probably experienced hardship. The average fuel value of one family's meals, for example, amounted to just 2,050 Cal/m/d, almost certainly a starvation ration in a community with no alternatives to manual labor. By comparison, the lowest level of energy consumption recorded in the town of Maryville exceeded 2,600 Cal/m/d.

In addition to lower energy intakes, winter dealt Georgia's mountain families a sharp setback in protein nutrition. Consumption for much of the year averaged slightly less than 100 g/m/d. Winter meals averaged just 84 g/m/d. That included only 9 g/m/d of animal protein. To some extent, cowpeas, a rich and complete source of protein and a frequent dish on Mountaineers' tables, must have helped make up for this. In any case, the Tallulah Falls area suffered from a high incidence of tuberculosis, a disease synergistically related to protein-calorie malnutrition.[24] Many residents of Crooked Creek also suffered from tuberculosis.[25]

MARYVILLE

Maryville, Tennessee, the Blount County seat, is situated in the foothills of the Great Smoky Mountains. Today it is a prosperous city of twenty-five thousand people, many of them employed at making aluminum and manufacturing automobile parts. Only four thousand people lived there when Professor Charles Wait began his study, but a railroad connection to Knoxville had been completed recently, and the town was growing.[26] Economic activity revolved around the lumber industry, with a few small factories and farms contributing as well. Local agriculture benefited from fertile valleys, and the hillsides around Maryville proved suitable for grazing livestock once they were cleared of timber.

Wait's study involved forty-four families. Some of them lived on the outskirts of town, and a few were located in the nearby mountains, but most resided in Maryville proper. The adult men earned their livings in a variety of

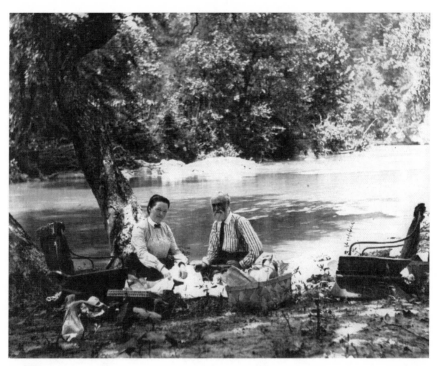

PHOTO 2.3
"Picnic" (1910). Couple likely from the Maryville area dining al fresco on a river bank.
(Courtesy of Growth of Democracy in Tennessee, a Grassroots Approach to Volunteer
Voices, http://idserver.utk.edu/?id=200600000001199, Blount County Public Library,
Maryville, TN [0020 000052 000203 0000].)

occupations. These included bricklayer, factory laborer, operating engineer, and railway-section hand. Wait inventoried the food supply of one farmer who doubled as a teacher and another who worked part time at a lumber mill. Women mainly occupied themselves as homemakers. Some took in washing or sewing; a few worked in factories. Several households had members who were unemployed.

Living conditions in Maryville were typical for small manufacturing towns throughout much of Appalachia. People resided in simple, mostly one-story structures. In or near town, frame buildings predominated. Plaster or paper usually covered the inside walls. The number of rooms varied, but few families had separate sitting or dining rooms. The living room ordinarily doubled as a sleeping room, and in some instances entire families bedded down in a single room. The rooms contained few furnishings. Clothes hung on nails in the walls. A handful of townspeople owned bureaus, center tables, and clocks. Some had curtains or shades for the windows, but most folks could afford nothing more than some beds, a few plain chairs, and a dining table covered with cotton or oilcloth. Families generally ate in the kitchen. Many had wood stoves for cooking, but these were not universal. Pantries were rare. People stored food in safes or kept it on open shelves. The kitchen often contained a table for washing dishes. Nobody, however, had plumbing.

House lots in Maryville normally afforded no more outdoor space than a small backyard. Steep slopes in some places precluded using this space to raise food, and in certain instances rental agreements prohibited it. Still, many Maryville residents grew vegetables for home use, and a few owned a fruit tree. Some families raised chickens. A few kept a horse, a cow, or a few pigs.

Wait spent nearly six months collecting dietaries around Maryville. The structure of a typical diet based on his data is outlined in table 2.3. Here we see the same core commodities that comprised the heart of Mountaineer fare—cured pork, milk, cornmeal, wheat flour, lard, butter, sugar, and potatoes—plus a number of other foods. These included beans, cabbage, and sweet potato, which were peripheral fare around Crooked Creek, as well as fresh beef and canned goods, victuals practically absent from that area.

Table 2.3. Typical Maryville Diet, Late Fall through Early Spring, 1901–1903

	Meat and Dairy	Grains and Dried Legumes	Fats, Oils, Sugars, and Starches	Roots and Tubers	Other Vegetables	Fruits and Misc.
Primary Core	salt pork buttermilk	cornmeal wheat flour	lard butter sugar	sweet potato	cabbage	
Secondary Core	fresh beef[1] pork sausage milk[2]	bean	molasses	potato	turnip	apple[3] peach[4]
Periphery	fresh pork[5] egg	cowpea	brown sugar		onion sauerkraut	blackberry[6]

1. mostly shoulder clod, shank, and round steak
2. both whole and skimmed
3. fresh and dried; also preserves
4. dried and canned
5. ribs and other cuts
6. canned and preserves

Most of Wait's inventories were conducted during the cold-weather months. This explains the presence of pork sausage and fresh beef among the core foods shown in table 2.3. Lower temperatures and diminished concerns about spoilage had the effect of increasing meat supplies. With the onset of winter, farmers everywhere began slaughtering hogs and other livestock. Coincidently, falling temperatures increased energy demands and stimulated people's interest in fat-rich products like pork sausage. Wait's data indicate that the contribution of animal fat to total energy intake increased steadily from October through December, began tapering off in January, and then rose again during March.

Maryville's diet disclosed a remarkable diversity around the edges, with a considerable number of foods appearing in less than 10 percent of the households. Animal products subsumed in this category included pig's head, pork liver, smoked ham, wild rabbit, perch, and canned sardines. Among the vegetables were parsnips, canned corn, peas, tomatoes, and gooseberries. Pickled beans, beets, and cucumbers were seen in some kitchens, and a few families purchased rice and rolled oats. Only two households purchased white bread.

Nutrition in Maryville in general was not good. Wait discovered underweight children in five households (over 10 percent of those studied). He estimated that nearly half of the families in his sample failed to supply adequate nourishment to every member.[27] Protein deficiency appeared to be widespread but unevenly distributed. The average consumption of animal-sourced protein in Maryville was 26 g/m/d during the winter and 22 g/m/d overall, but half of the families involved in Wait's study consumed less than 18 g/m/d. He speculated that protein deficiency first became a hazard among Mountaineers after prior generations hunted to exhaustion the large game species that once populated the area.[28] As with protein, so with energy. Twenty-six families (60 percent of those studied) fell below the average level of energy intake. Ten families consumed less than 3,000 Cal/m/d. One hundred years ago, a man toiling twelve hours a day milling wood or shoveling gravel would have needed approximately 3,500 Cal/m/d to stay healthy and keep his job. Furthermore, the breadwinner had to come first if there was to be any food on the table. This left the mother (particularly if she was not a wage earner) and children too young to work vulnerable. Likely they would go hungry if there was not enough food to go around. This exposure, all too common in certain parts of the world today, probably accounted for Maryville's underweight children.

IMPERFECTLY SKILLED MECHANICS

Three dietaries from Knoxville, Tennessee, collected by Charles Wait, and one from Athens, Georgia, compiled by H. C. White, provide a glimpse of food consumption in urban households situated just beyond the Land of Do Without.[29] This is a tiny sample, to be sure, but enough to sketch the eating habits among working-class families on the economically developed edges of Appalachia and show how they differed from those of the mountains.

The families represented in this set of studies can be characterized as economically secure but barely so. White characterized the family he studied in Athens as one of "imperfectly skilled mechanics, quite typical of a somewhat numerous class of white people in this section."[30] "Imperfectly skilled" translates to "semi-skilled" in modern parlance. The term *mechanic* referred to anyone who worked with hand tools. In this case, the men of the family—a father and two sons—worked as carpenters. Wait's Knoxville studies concerned the diets of three families supported by hard-working mechanics.

Together these inventories revealed a core diet of sixteen foods. These included the core foods typical of the Land of Do Without with the addition of various cuts of fresh pork, a variety of fresh fish, eggs, rice, cowpeas, syrup, and greens. Several meats, including lamb, smoked pork, bologna, smoked fish, and chicken, held peripheral places in the diet. Other peripherals included oat flakes, oatmeal, crackers, tapioca, canned corn, canned tomatoes, fruit jellies, and raisins.

Table 2.2 presents an estimate of what the urban working-class meals offered nutritionally. It shows high protein values, especially on the animal side, compared to Crooked Creek, northeastern Georgia, and Maryville. A hefty portion of the food budget (an average of 64 percent) was spent on meat and dairy products. This strong budgetary commitment to meat and dairy goods helps explain why families took in more energy from animal sources than all other foods combined.

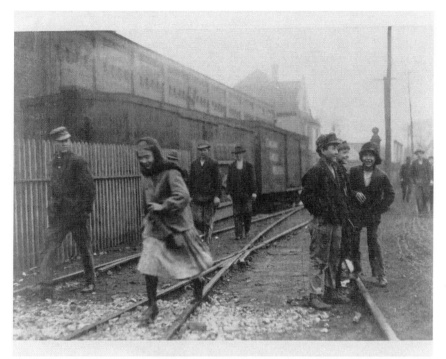

PHOTO 2.4
"Noon Hour Brookside Cotton Mills . . ." (1910). Knoxville workers, including several youngsters, take a break; most employees carried their lunch to the mill. (Photograph by Lewis Wickes Hine. Courtesy of the records of the National Child Labor Committee [LC-DIG-nclc-02026], U.S. Library of Congress, Prints and Photographs Division.)

SOUTHERN STUDENTS

Chapter 6 looks at student diets in some detail. Suffice it to say here that in addition to working-class dietaries for Knoxville and Athens, we have six student dietaries, five conducted by Wait in various dining halls at the University of Tennessee and one carried out by White at the University of Georgia.[31] We can take these as middle- to upper-class dietaries because at the time, higher education was normally beyond the reach of working-class families.

The diet of southern students, as modeled from Wait and White's food inventories, was at once rural and cosmopolitan. At its core, there is nothing to suggest that higher education did anything to dislodged fundamental southern tastes. Students exhibited no less commitment to salt pork, lard, cornmeal, and molasses than the poorest Mountaineers. At the same time, however,

RECIPE 2.2

CHOW-CHOW

The presence of chow-chow on the table of an eating club at the University of Tennessee in 1896 provides a good example of cosmopolitan influence on campus culture. Chinese immigrants introduced chow-chow to the United States and initiated its cross-country diffusion.[1] The dish first reached the Appalachians sometime in the 1890s. It eventually became a regional favorite.[2]

Chow-chow can be described best as a relish based on a variety of garden products. It provided a ready answer to the question of how to save the odds and ends from the vegetable patch before the first frost: pickle and can them. Chow-chow in Appalachia usually contains green tomato, cabbage, and onion, but after that just about anything goes. A batch might contain some red tomato, apple, celery, corn, cucumber, green beans, and a variety of peppers.

Historian Mark Sohn provides a quick, overnight recipe for chow-chow that captures its essential flavors.[3] His recipe calls for one cup of cabbage or one green tomato, one bell pepper, one medium onion, one small cucumber, one tablespoon of salt, one-fourth cup of sugar, one teaspoon of ground mustard, one-half teaspoon of turmeric, one-third cup of white vinegar, and one-third cup of water. The first step involves chopping the raw vegetables into small pieces and combining them in a bowl. Measure four cups of the combined vegetables into another bowl and mix with the salt. Let this mixture stand for most of the day or overnight. Then drain the mixture and add the mustard, turmeric, vinegar, and water. Simmer for fifteen minutes. The chow-chow can be served hot or cold, and it can be used as a condiment, garnish, or vegetable dish.

A recipe for chow-chow can found in nearly every book of American recipes published during the Gilded Age. Juliet Corson's recipe, published in 1885, was typical:

Remove the defective and green outer leaves of firm white cabbages, and shave enough to fill a four-quart measure; measure an equal quantity each of green tomatoes, small green cucumbers, and green peppers, and slice them thin, after wiping them with a wet cloth; put them into earthen or wooden vessels, sprinkling a pint of salt among them; let them stand over night; drain them the next day, put them into a preserving-kettle with a pint of small red peppers and the following spices: one ounce each of whole mace, peppercorns, mustard-seed, and powdered turmeric; half an ounce each of whole cloves, celery-seed, and grated horseradish; and sufficient vinegar to cover them; boil them gently for half an hour, and then cool them, and put them up in earthen or glass jars with close covers.[4]

Nowadays, for the sake of food safety, cooks pack their chow-chow in ringed jars and process them in a hot water bath for fifteen minutes. A traditional chow-chow like Corson's mellowed for a week or two before serving.

NOTES

1. See Charles E. Wait, *Nutritional Investigations at the University of Tennessee in 1896 and 1897*, U.S. Department of Agriculture Office of Experiment Stations Bulletin 53 (Washington, DC: U.S. Government Printing Office, 1898), 20.

2. Mark F. Sohn, *Appalachian Home Cooking History, Culture, and Recipes* (Lexington: University of Kentucky Press, 2005), 53.

3. Ibid., 217–18.

4. Juliet Corson, *Miss Corson's Practical American Cookery and Household Management* (New York: Dodd, Mead, 1885), 260.

college dining facilities offered items not ordinarily found in most areas of the South and certainly not in the mountains of Tennessee and Georgia. There was the fresh beef eaten in southern towns and cities, but veal was also part of the diet. Students' meals also included commercially baked bread and dishes made with macaroni. Campus cooks worked with Graham flour, a product regarded as a healthier alternative to white flour. Menus featured more fruits and vegetables than normally encountered in southern working-class households. The presence of cranberries, lemons, and bananas on college tables clearly attested to cosmopolitan influences.

Table 2.2 reports the average nutritional contents of college diets. From a comparative perspective, they contained about 10 percent less energy than working-class diets and about 30 percent less animal fat. While working-class householders were taking more than 50 percent of their energy from animal sources on average, meat and dairy contributed little more than 40 percent of the energy consumed by students. Compared to mechanics, students, on average, spent a considerably smaller fraction of their food budget on animal products, but for both the costs were about the same (approximately ten cents per day). Also on a par was the consumption of animal-derived protein but only because of considerable waste on the students' part. Generally speaking, they purchased higher-quality meats than members of the working class; consequently, protein consumption ought to have been higher. Yet students consigned to the garbage over a quarter of the meat protein they purchased.

THE NUTRITION TRANSITION

Diet and nutrition throughout history have undergone a series of alterations defined by patterns of food use and corresponding health problems. These changes have picked up speed over the past two centuries.[32] Nowadays, the nutrition transition accompanying modern economic development seems to occur almost overnight. Developing regions typically experience a sharp increase in noncommunicable diseases associated with overnutrition. This comes as a shock because just a few years before the problem had been undernutrition. Back then, occupations were labor intensive, and people consumed monotonous, starchy diets that were high in fiber and low in fat. Authorities fretted over low birth weights, undernourished and sickly children, seasonal hunger, and occasionally famine. Economic development ushered in commercial foods, thereby paving the way to big increases in the consumption of refined grains and foods derived from animals. These tend to be low in fiber and high in total fat, saturated fat, sugar, and salt, contributing substantially to overweight and obesity and, in due course, to diabetes, hypertension, and mortality related to cardiovascular disease.

Although we have no systematic medical records for southern Appalachia a century ago and cannot talk about the incidence of disease, the historical data strongly suggest a nutrition transition in progress. Comparing the various diets considered in this chapter uncovers the process in cross-section, as it were, with Crooked Creek and the Tallulah Falls area, in effect representing the predevelopment stage of the transition. Here the staple was a minimally processed cornmeal that contributed most of the populations' food energy. Yet in both communities diet lacked variety and consisted of only about half a dozen foods over the course of a week. In a developing industrial town like Maryville, where commercially canned and other processed foods were available, the average number of foods per week for winter and spring increased slightly. If we look to Crooked Creek as a baseline, it would appear that the consumption of refined wheat flour increased in Maryville at the expense of crude cornmeal, and the proportion of energy drawn from vegetable products declined. Semi-skilled mechanics' families in Knoxville and Athens relied much less on vegetable sources as a proportion of total energy consumption, but at the same time their diets were more varied than the diets of Mountaineers. More varied still were the diets at the most metropolitan end of this continuum. Here the most affluent group of student boarders purchased no less than fifty-seven commodities in order to prepare the dishes that members ate over the course of a week.

Much of the variety in the diet of students can be attributed to their taste for fruits and vegetables. Deep in the mountains, folks ate Irish potatoes and sweet potatoes. Other than that, vegetable consumption was negligible, especially in Crooked Creek, where only two types of vegetables—cabbages and onions—were served in more than 10 percent of the households. Georgia's Mountaineers ate considerable quantities of cabbage and apples, especially during the winter. All told, six fruits and vegetables were at least peripheral to the diet around Tallulah Falls. Maryville's residents commonly ate about the same number of these foods. Working-class households in the Knoxville and Athens studies consumed eleven fruits and vegetables in addition to potatoes. On campus, potatoes included potato chips, but the number of other fruits and vegetables jumped to thirty. However, while variety increased, grams per day generally decreased. With northeastern Georgia's winter dietaries as a baseline, fruit consumption decreased from 177 g/m/d to 93 g/m/d in Maryville to 71 g/m/d among the urban working class to 48 g/m/d among university students. Vegetable consumption decreased from 337 g/m/d to 302 g/m/d in town to 215 g/m/d among university students.[33]

Transitioning from a hunger-prone society to a society subject to the afflictions of overeating has always been coincident with eating more foods from animal sources, and the pattern in and around the southern Appalachians was no exception. Neither Wait nor White found much meat eating in their collections of dietaries from remote mountain communities. Wait declared the diet of Crooked Creek's inhabitants as "practically vegetarian."[34] Cured pork was universally consumed, of course, but out of seventy-four households, one finds beef listed for only seventeen, fish for just two, and poultry for none. Only eight dietaries listed eggs. Small game animals may have been inventoried more often in Crooked Creek had Wait undertook his research a little later in the year. The chief dairy product in the mountains was buttermilk, which was tallied for thirty-four households. Whole milk was counted fourteen times. By contrast, the scientists noted beef in three of the four working-class kitchens they visited and in all of the boarding clubs. Fish was popular among mechanics and students alike. Two-thirds of the campus dietaries listed poultry, and everyone in town ate eggs. In addition, every urban working-class household and student boarding club consumed whole milk as well as buttermilk.

All told, this made urban diets rich in fat compared to the diets of Mountaineers. Indeed, while upland residents, including those living in Maryville, were drawing somewhere around 30 percent their energy from fat, the average for urban working-class households was close to 50 percent. Again taking the remote villages as our predevelopment baseline, we see that the contribution of food from plant sources to the total energy supply decreased from upward of 67 percent to about 60 percent in Maryville to less than 45 percent in urban working-class households. Conversely, dependence on animal fat as a source of energy, and, by proxy, the level of saturated fats in the diet, increased from as little as 21 percent among mountain dwellers to more than twice that in mechanics' households. Students showed somewhat less enthusiasm for meat products and animal fat than skilled and semi-skilled laborers, something nutritionists would regard as typical of educated communities in the postdevelopment phase of the nutrition transition. Yet the great irony is that while university students backed away from meat and fat and consumed more fruits and vegetables, their intake of animal fat still far exceeded the level documented in the backwoods. The Mountaineers' "frontier diet" was once depicted by foods swimming in grease.[35] In truth, metropolitan communities have come to prefer their fats and oils well hidden but in quantities much greater than yesteryear's.

3

African Americans and Soul Foods

Soul food represents a cooking style originated by African American slaves out of necessity.[1] The problem was cotton and other cash crops and the way they rendered food production to a kind of afterthought. In many parts of the South, slaves produced much of their own food. With little time available to see to their own needs, they concentrated on vegetables that were easy to grow and store. Their meats were coarse and fatty, not by choice, but because of their masters' begrudging attitude and chronic penny-pinching. Offcuts of meat, offal, and other cheap foods continued to dominate the African American bill of fare after slavery because most families could not afford "to live high on the hog." Yet black people remained undaunted. They made up for their rough and simple cuisine with a loving attitude in the kitchen and an open-handed generosity with whatever food they had.

Today's soul food harks back to those earlier times. Much of its richness as a cuisine stems from its pork specialties. Chitterlings or chitlins (intestines of hogs slow cooked and often eaten with vinegar and hot sauce), cracklings (fried pork skin), fatback (salted pork fat, generally used to season vegetables), ham hocks, hog jowls (sliced and usually cooked with chitlins), souse (made from pig snouts, lips, and ears), pigs' feet (sometimes pickled), and ribs rank among the most famous. Country fried steak (beef dredged in seasoned flour and deep fried), beef neck bones, fried chicken (with cornmeal or seasoned flour breading), and fried fish (often dredged in cornmeal) also count as mainstays. As for vegetables, soul food menus feature black-eyed peas, lima beans, okra (fried or stewed), red beans, and sweet potatoes (sometimes called yams in the United States). Other classics include biscuits, chow-chow (a spicy pickle relish using a variety of vegetables), cornbread, grits, hot sauce (cayenne peppers, vinegar, and spices), rice, sorghum, and watermelon.

Nutritionists consider a diet heavy on soul foods unhealthy.[2] Concerns arise primarily from the common convention of cooking and seasoning with pork fat and because so many dishes are fried, usually in lard or hydrogenated vegetable oil. These practices produce dishes packed with energy and dripping with trans fatty acids. "Trans fats," as they are often called, arise from the process of hydrogenating unsaturated oils. This causes them to become solid and act like saturated fats. Trans fats raise the level of low-density lipoprotein ("bad cholesterol") in the blood and increase the risk of coronary heart disease. They also decrease levels of high-density lipoprotein that helps remove cholesterol from arteries. All told, a steady diet of soul food without significant exercise leads to disproportionately high occurrences of obesity, hypertension, cardiac and circulatory problems, and diabetes, all too often resulting in early death.

The dangers notwithstanding, many African Americans think of soul food as comfort food. It calls to mind family and friends and, in keeping with its name, is supposed to feed the spirit as well as the body. People regard it as part of their ancestral heritage and as an emblem of ethnic identity. Soul food restaurants ranging from chicken shacks to upscale clubs exist all across the nation, and in big cities with large black populations, one finds them in especially large numbers.

This was not the case around 1900, when researchers studied food consumption among African Americans in New York, Philadelphia, and Washington, DC. Dietaries showed blacks eating sweet potatoes in such places, but otherwise soul foods were scarcely seen. Nevertheless, projects in the areas of the South succeeded in documenting several diets prototypical of modern soul food.[3] This chapter recounts these traditions and examines their relationships to geography and commerce. It compares African American diets across a rural-urban continuum reaching from remote regions of Alabama and eastern Virginia into metropolitan areas of the Northeast. The progressive expansion and improvement of diet along this continuum and the absence of soul foods at the metropolitan end appears to have been a response to available alternatives in the marketplace and a result of rational choices on the part of black consumers.

TUSKEGEE AND THE BLACK BELT

Of the thousands of southern towns and villages dedicated to cotton culture and otherwise well qualified to host the OES's first look at African American food habits, W. O. Atwater and his staff picked Tuskegee, Alabama, home of Booker T. Washington and the Tuskegee Normal and Industrial Institute. Destined to become one of the country's foremost schools of higher education for blacks, the institute was only four years old at this point, but already its principal was a respected figure among educators and well on his way to becoming nationally influential on matters of race. Atwater regarded Washington as a trustworthy collaborator. He had no trouble convincing him of the value of dietary studies. Washington gladly accepted Atwater's offer of a research appointment, but H. M. Smith was dispatched from OES headquarters to take care of the actual work.

Smith did not work alone, however. He began fieldwork in the spring of 1895 assisted by J. W. Hoffman, a Tuskegee resident and member of the institute's staff. Smith and Hoffman completed their observations in June 1895, but Hoffman undertook another round on his own in December. He continued working through February 1896 in order to capture winter eating habits. The institute's farm manager recruited subjects for both phases of the project. All told, he enlisted the cooperation of eighteen families, including his own.

These subjects represented a range of social and economic conditions. Several families resided in Tuskegee proper. Most, however, were tenant farmers and plantation workers, some living as far as nine miles away from the village. Those in or near Tuskegee lived in relative comfort, especially if they were attached to the institute. Others, particularly folks employed on large plantations, lived in hopeless poverty and were typical of the majority of African Americans inhabiting the so-called Black Belt, a fertile plain stretching approximately 300 miles (480 kilometers) across central Alabama and northeastern Mississippi.

The Black Belt's African Americans for the most part were members of a rural proletariat or working class. Around Tuskegee, most rented between twenty and sixty acres of land and worked it behind their own mule or ox. Many families owned at least one pig and several chickens. Those living in and near the village usually kept a cow. People dedicated most of their land to cotton, their cash crop. For food, they grew corn, sweet potatoes, sugar cane, and sorghum, though rarely did anyone raise enough of these commodities to meet their own family's needs year round. To make matters worse, only a few households kept kitchen gardens for raising collards, turnips, and other vegetables.

Cotton's prior claim on people's time and energy applied to every man, woman, and child strong enough to lift a hoe. Planting began in March and ran through June. It demanded an all-out effort at the same time of year that farmers might otherwise be planting subsistence crops. Then came picking, with another round of labor just as intense. It got under way in mid-August

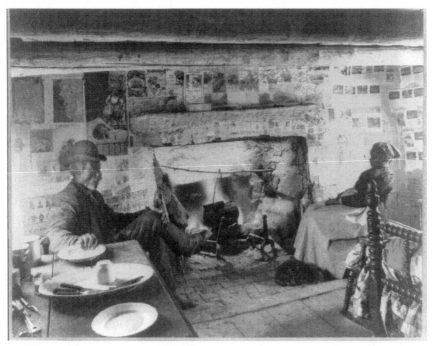

PHOTO 3.1
"African American Couple Sitting in One-Room Cabin near Fireplace" (c. 1900). Cooking pot hangs over the fire; dinnerware is on the table. (Photograph by Geo. S. Cook. Courtesy of Miscellaneous Items [LC-USZ62-28021], U.S. Library of Congress, Prints and Photographs Division.)

and continued through November. In between planting and picking came a "laying-by time." This midsummer interlude for resting up, visiting family and friends, and attending camp meetings extended over a period of four or five weeks. Tenants and plantation hands normally spent the winter doing little or nothing. A few collected wood and sold it. Some repaired fences. Others made chairs or baskets, but hardly anybody found wage work.

Tenant housing throughout the region consisted mainly of one- or two-room log cabins meagerly furnished. Family members generally possessed a couple of rope bedsteads, a few corn-shuck mattresses, and some patchwork quilts. Here and there someone owned a clock, but more often than not it failed to keep time. Typical household objects included a cupboard, an assortment of dishes, and a wooden chest or perhaps an old trunk for keeping food and clothing. In addition, there was usually a pine table, several chairs, a pair of andirons, and an iron pot. Few rural residents owned a cooking stove.

The women of the house usually prepared meals in front of a fireplace, relying on lard, cornmeal, molasses, and pieces of salt pork as staples. Table 3.1 shows these foods as the core components of the Tuskegee diet. The table also identifies wheat flour as a core item, but only recently had it become cheap enough to use on a regular basis. The biscuit was still a newcomer to local tables at the height of the Gilded Age. The cured pork was a long-standing favorite, but by the 1890s it was no longer a local or even a regional product. Instead, in cabin after cabin Smith and Hoffman saw commercially

Table 3.1. Typical Winter–Spring Diet, Tuskegee, 1895–1896

	Meat and Dairy	Grains and Dried Legumes	Fats, Oils, Sugars, and Starches	Roots and Tubers	Other Vegetables	Fruits and Misc.
Primary Core	bacon	cornmeal wheat flour	lard sugar molasses			
Secondary Core	fresh pork[1] milk buttermilk		butter	sweet potato	greens[2]	
Periphery	egg	rice cowpea				

1. various cuts
2. types not specified

packed bacon from Chicago. They seldom came across lean pork. The very term *meat* meant fatty pork in Tuskegee. Some locals claimed that they were unfamiliar with any other sort of meat except chicken and wild species such as possum and rabbit.[4]

Area families generally cooked the same simple meals day after day. Preparations began by placing a thin slice of bacon or salt pork in a frying pan and mixing cornmeal and water to make a dough. This was plunked onto a skillet or the flat surface of a hoe. The skillet or the hoe, along with the frying pan, was positioned over a fire for ten or fifteen minutes. By then, the dough had baked and the pork was fried crisp. For a finishing touch, some molasses might be mixed into the leftover grease to make "sap." It served as a kind of gravy to accompany the cornbread or "hoe cake."

Now and again families had other things to eat. "Crackling bread" was made by frying fat until it was crisp; crushing it into a mixture of cornmeal, water, soda, and salt; and then baking it like ordinary cornbread. Collards or turnips were boiled with pork fat to give the vegetables a "rich taste." Those who owned a cow used its milk to make a watery butter. It was churned in little clay vessels called splashers. Members of the household ate the butter fresh and had a little buttermilk to drink most of the year. Sometimes during late autumn or winter, fresh pork and sweet potatoes might be served, and every so often someone prepared a possum. The cook, on such occasions, seasoned the carcass with red peppers and baked it surrounded by sweet potatoes in a big pot.

The Tuskegee inventories indicated that vegetables other than sweet potatoes were peripheral to the diet of most residents. Only the unspecified greens listed in table 3.1 showed up in an appreciable number of dietaries. The researchers came across collards only once. Every other vegetable they tallied, including beets, cabbage, green corn, okra, onions, string beans, and tomatoes, was found exclusively in but one household—the home of the institute's farm manager. His family's use of dried apples and strawberries and the consumption of blackberries and peaches by another family associated with the institute accounted for all of the fruits identified in the study.

Other disparities existed between families connected to the institute and every other household enrolled in the study. Institute families were singular

RECIPE 3.1

ROASTED POSSUM

This recipe comes from *Dishes and Beverages of the Old South*, by Martha McCulloch-Williams.[1] Not many readers will have an opportunity, let alone the inclination, to prepare this dish, but read the instructions anyway. The recipe relates in detail what went into the making of the very same roast mentioned in the Tuskegee dietaries.

McCulloch-Williams, a white person, learned southern cooking as a child, seated on the biscuit block in her family's detached kitchen, some thirty yards out behind the house. There her "mammy," although a black woman and a slave, ruled. She worked throughout the day, fixing meals for the McCulloch family. She often followed her own recipes and served dishes informed by the African American tastes and traditions that she had embraced from the time she was a little girl.

McCulloch-Williams proffered just a few game recipes in *Dishes and Beverages.* She instructed her readers on how to barbecue rabbit and squirrel, how to make quail pie, and how to roast a wild duck. She went into the most detail describing how to roast a possum:

> Chill thoroughly after scraping and drawing. Save all the inside fat, let it soak in weak salt water until cooking time, then rinse it well, and partly try [fry?] it out in the pan before putting in the **possum**. Unless he is huge, leave him whole, skewering him flat, and laying him skin side up in the pan. Set in a hot oven and cook until crisply tender, taking care there is no scorching. Roast a dozen good sized sweet potatoes—in ashes if possible, if not, bake them covered in a deep pan. Peel when done, and lay while hot around the **possum**, turning them over and over in the abundant gravy. He should have been lightly salted when hung up, and fully seasoned, with salt, pepper, and a trifle of mustard, when put down to cook. Dish him in a big platter,

(continued)

RECIPE 3.1 (*continued*)

lay the potatoes, which should be partly browned, around him, add a
little boiling water to the pan, shake well around, and pour the gravy
over everything. Hot corn bread, strong black coffee, or else sharp
cider, and very hot sharp pickles are the things to serve with him.[2]

NOTES

1. Martha McCulloch-Williams, *Dishes and Beverages of the Old South*
(New York: McBride Nast, 1913).

2. Ibid., 175–76.

---

in their use of chicken and mutton, and with but one exception, the families of
institute employees accounted for all of the beef consumption reported. In addition, the diets of institute families were twice as varied as those of ordinary
farmers. Some farm families subsisted on just four commodities for the entire
two weeks they were observed.

The underlying problem was that tenants and plantation hands all across
the Black Belt remained in a kind of bondage many decades after emancipation. Instead of frank slavery, African Americans in Alabama labored
throughout the Gilded Age under a form of debt peonage locally referred to
as "the mortgage system." Landowners under this arrangement made loans
to tenants, which enabled them to buy seed, tools, and provisions sufficient
to last the growing season. Tenants in return signed a "waive note," giving
lenders first right to whatever portion of the crop they needed in order to
settle the debt. With high rates of interest, a tenant had little cotton left to
sell after the landlord took his share. Even a tenant who made good money
on a crop had to subsist for a time on scant rations because more often than
not savings were spent by February. In the meantime, households exhausted
whatever corn and molasses they had in store and had to rely all the more
heavily on purchased provisions until they sapped their credit. At this point,

family members had to go hungry and wait until the following spring when, once again, credit became available (see chapter 4).

EASTERN VIRGINIA

The OES followed up its Alabama study with two projects in eastern Virginia. The first looked into the eating habits of black families settled in the Great Dismal Swamp of Franklin County.[5] The second dealt with families in Elizabeth City County and the city of Hampton, a Chesapeake Bay port on the north side of Hampton Roads.[6] Hampton Normal and Agricultural Institute (today's Hampton University), a U.S. land-grant school dedicated to the education of African and Native Americans, sponsored both inquiries.

H. B. Frissell, principal of the institute, compiled the Franklin County dietaries. The venture seemed destined to fail at first. Recruiting subjects and weighing their foods required traveling back and forth every day through a malaria-infested area seldom visited by outsiders. The unusual comings and goings alarmed local whites and provoked outcries against the project. Frissell responded with patient explanations and eventually calmed their fears.[7]

Frissell's research, which took place during the spring of 1897, involved twelve families. They lived near their cultivations in tiny cabins on small tracts of rented land. Dwellings typically were built of boards and equipped with a fireplace. This was often a family's sole source of light as well as heat. Few of the swamp's inhabitants could afford to purchase lamp oil or candles.

The farmers cultivated the swamplands by creating "dead-tree farms." These were started on forested plots by girdling the trees and removing the underbrush. This established a clearing littered with dead tree trunks. Cotton, peanuts, sweet potatoes, and other crops were planted amid the debris. Farmers produced most of their own food in this way. Landlords customarily collected rents in commodities, sometimes as much as half of the crop. The swamp dwellers supplemented their agricultural efforts with earnings from odd jobs. Compensation came in the form of "rations" rather than money. As a result, a number of families never needed to purchase supplies from the store. Some patronized it occasionally but only to purchase a few cents worth of salt. Others bought canned goods and small quantities of baking powder, green coffee or tea, and vinegar.

Frissell characterized the local diet as "hog and hominy." As in Tuskegee, the bulk of it consisted of cornmeal that was mixed with water and baked. In the Dismal Swamp, the cornmeal included a considerable amount of bran, and the water was usually brackish and muddy. The finished product was called "ash cake" because the dough was inserted directly into the hot ashes of the fireplace to bake. On the hog side, Franklin County's blacks enjoyed more variety than folks around Tuskegee. In addition to belly bacon and lard as components of the core diet, people had salt sides (side bacon) and boiled pork shoulders. Fresh fish was another favorite. Sweet potatoes, cabbage, and mustard greens came to the table regularly, frequently accompanied by a bit of smoked or salted herring for extra flavor. Peripheral springtime foods included ham, pork sausage, pork jowl, eggs, milk, brown sugar, molasses, collard sprouts, dried apples, strawberries, canned tomatoes, and canned peaches. Families dined on frogs, turtles, and snakes at certain times of the year. Frissell's notebooks also listed fresh beef (both flank and shoulder), dried beef, beef liver, pork liver, chitterlings, haslet (meatloaf from pork offal), chicken, eel, white bread, sponge cake, canned blackberries, and various pickles.

Atwater asked a student, Isabel Bevier, to collect the Elizabeth City County and Hampton dietaries.[8] These were places culturally unlike the Great Dismal Swamp. Indeed, if we take Frissell's Franklin County households to approximate a folk community, Bevier's sample represented a more metropolitan way of life. Nearly everyone in the Elizabeth City–Hampton area was immersed in commerce and industry. Many blacks had small plots of land on which they raised two crops a year. Early vegetables were shipped north. Later in the season, growers dispatched potatoes, peas, sweet corn, and various fruits to Washington, DC, and other nearby markets. Besides this truck farming, African Americans held jobs in the local fishing industry and in the shipyards at Newport News, Virginia. In Hampton, they pursued a variety of trades and professions, and they owned a number of local businesses.

Bevier conducted three of her dietaries in Hampton and four in rural areas of the county during the spring of 1898. Two of the families in town lived in large, well-furnished homes. The others resided in small frame houses. The walls inside were covered with newspaper, and the furniture frequently consisted of no more than a couple of chairs, a bench, a table, and a cupboard. Less often, there was a stove. About the half of the people in the county owned

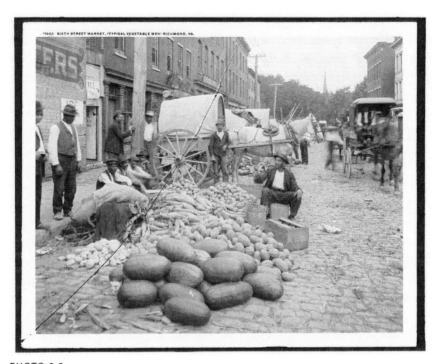

PHOTO 3.2
"Sixth Street Market (Typical Vegetable Men), Richmond, Va." (1908?). African American truck farmers provisioned the towns and cities throughout the Tidewater region. (Courtesy of the Detroit Publishing Company Photograph Collection [LC-D401-71020], U.S. Library of Congress, Prints and Photographs Division.)

a cow. Most kept chickens and a pig and raised vegetables such as corn, sweet potato, and cabbage in small gardens.

Consumption patterns reflected Hampton's location and commercial orientation. Not unexpectedly, fresh fish was a primary constituent in the local diet. Pork was consumed as frequently, however, and in greater quantities. Families fortunate enough to own a pig killed it in December and ate it over the course of the winter, but most people had to content themselves with "white meat," a local euphemism for salt pork shipped from Chicago. County residents also purchased various forms of commercially processed beef. Indeed, smoked, chipped, and corned beef combined counted as another primary component in the typical diet. Bacon, ham, and chicken were secondary.

Dairy products were peripheral. This was because most milk got churned into butter and traded at local shops for other provisions. The butter making took place in a box-like structure referred to locally as "the dairy." It stood near the house, about two feet above the ground on wooden legs. From the dairy, the by-product of the churn, the buttermilk, went to the children. The butter itself was exchanged for cornmeal, wheat flour, rice, granulated sugar, and cabbage. White bread was also popular, and since most families did not own an oven, it was mainly store bought. Still, there were those who disdained commercially baked bread and avoided it entirely. Bevier found that biscuits and hoe cakes led the way as the two most popular kinds of bread.

URBAN COMMUNITIES

Ellen Richards and Amelia Shapleigh's Philadelphia dietaries, S. E. Foreman's Washington budgetaries, and Alfred Hess and Lester Unger's nutritional research in New York City introduce us to the food habits of African Americans living in densely populated urban communities. Carried out in 1892 and intended to assess the nutrition of the various ethnicities served by a local settlement house, Richards and Shapleigh's work recorded the eating habits of five African American households.[9] Foreman, who tabulated the expenses of nineteen impoverished households during both summer and winter in 1905 and 1906, identified two of his cases as African American.[10]

We have only bits of information about the groups that took part in these studies. Richards and Shapleigh's notes identified two of the households that they studied as childless. The others contained as many as five children. Adult women outnumbered adult men by more than two to one. One of Forman's African American households consisted of an elderly rag picker, his wife, and three children. The other, headed by a flour-mill worker and his wife, contained five children. The rag picker brought home about five dollars a week. His wife took in washing. Each week she earned an additional two or three dollars. This family occupied four rooms with no running water in a two-story frame building located in an alley. The flour-mill employee earned nine dollars a week. His wife, too, did laundry to help make ends meet. The family rented a two-story frame house containing four small rooms and no toilet.

Table 3.2 combines the Philadelphia dietaries and Washington budgetaries in order to represent a typical African American urban diet for the cold-weather months. Here the absence of cured pork, cornmeal, and lard from the core diet signaled unequivocally a table very different from that set in black

Table 3.2. Typical Winter Diet, Poor African Americans, Philadelphia and Washington, DC, 1892–1906

	Meat and Dairy	Grains and Dried Legumes	Fats, Oils, Sugars, and Starches	Roots and Tubers	Other Vegetables	Fruits and Misc.
Primary Core	fresh beef[1] milk	white bread	butter sugar	potato sweet potato		
Secondary Core	pork sausage	rice bean			cabbage	
Periphery	fresh pork[2] ham bacon pudding[3] fresh mutton[4] sheep liver chicken fresh fish[5] egg	wheat flour oatmeal cornmeal scrapple hominy bun pie[6] cake[7]	lard	onion	canned tomato	apple

1. different cuts but mainly shoulder
2. assorted cuts
3. pork and possibly other meat
4. chops and a variety of other cuts
5. variety of species
6. unspecified types
7. unspecified types

communities further south. With whole milk replacing buttermilk as a core item, and with beef, white bread, and potatoes as staples, the diet outlined here appears to have been not much different from the diet of poor whites, save for the presence of sweet potatoes. The near absence of green vegetables from the table represented a seasonal artifact. Foreman's summer budgetaries listed kale, spinach, spurrey, and string beans. Both of his subjects switched from cornmeal to wheat flour for the summer, but they continued to eat potatoes, sweet potatoes, and cabbage throughout the year.

In the fall of 1916 and the winter of 1917, Alfred Hess and Lester Unger measured the food consumption of African American mothers in New York City.[11] Their purpose was to discover the causes of rickets in children. The two investigators suspected (wrongly) that the central problem was maternal nutrition. Research to test their hypothesis focused on the Columbus Hill area of the city, where the incidence of the disease was especially high. Most of the residents of the neighborhood were black, and most came from the West Indies.

Hess and Unger did not publish a detailed listing of foods consumed by the women they studied. They reported that most women ate either meat or fish daily, accompanied by rice or potatoes. Fruits and other vegetables were eaten, on average, twice a week, except during late autumn and winter. The consumption of fresh vegetables during that part of the year fell to about once every ten days.

The researchers offered almost no information about the children's food consumption. However, we know now that rickets in children usually involves a deficiency of vitamin D in their diets and that the disease was an especially serious problem among blacks. The reason is that vitamin D is produced by skin stimulated by ultraviolet rays, normally from the sun. Dark skin impedes the process. When dark-skinned people reside in northern latitudes and other places that receive scant sunlight, the situation can be dangerous. Around the time that Hess and Unger were conducting their inquiry, an estimated 80 percent of all infants in Boston showed signs of rickets. Studies of the disease in New Haven, Connecticut, and New Orleans, Louisiana, found it to be widespread, especially among African Americans.[12]

Few foods other than fish offer plenty of vitamin D. Liver, which happens to be a good source, has never been popular in the United States. Yet it does show up in table 3.2. Taking Philadelphia alone, sheep's liver counted as a core food. Settlement workers may have recommended it to anxious parents. Maybe feeding it to children regularly was a matter of folk knowledge. Whatever the case, liver's salience suggests that African American households were actively addressing the threat of rickets in at least one urban area.

THE INSTITUTE FOR COLORED YOUTH

The Institute for Colored Youth (now known as Cheyney University of Pennsylvania) may have stood amid a rustic landscape, but it was an institution committed to the most modern and progressive ideas of the early twentieth century. This was exemplified in a nutritional context in 1906, when the administration found itself no longer able to find suppliers willing to provision the school's kitchen at wholesale prices.[13] The problem was not enough students. This left administrators facing the prospect of having to feed sixty boarding students with nutritious and affordable meals while paying retail for the ingredients.

School officials addressed their predicament aggressively. Staff members kept a watchful eye over the storeroom, kitchen, and dining room. They received instructions to measure everything and to exercise the strictest economies from the initial purchase to the final disposal. Faculty members integrated cost reduction into the domestic science curriculum, and they engaged the entire student body in finding ways to reduce expenses. These endeavors paid off. By the end of the 1907–1908 school year, the cost of feeding a Cheyney student had been pared to twenty-one cents a day.

To celebrate, the administration proudly published a dining hall dietary for the month of October and daily menus for the entire school year.[14] These show that school officials, in spite of their zeal for cost cutting, did not saddle students with dreary and unappetizing meals. Throughout the drive to reduce costs, students received plenty of meat (especially cuts of fresh beef), milk, butter, bread, and potatoes. These standard components of the core diet were supplemented with fresh fish, mutton or lamb, rice, and tomatoes nearly every month. Other items came and went. Apples, primary in October, disappeared by January. Eggs, hardly seen in October, became a core food in April. Such changes reflected seasonal availabilities and prices. Other switches, such as the sudden appearance of a generic breakfast cereal as a core item of the diet in July, may have been opportunistic—a good price for whatever reason at the time. During the month of October, the kitchen used more than ninety-five different commodities. Weekly menus listed approximately seventy distinct dishes. Most of the recipes came from Fannie Farmer's *Boston Cooking-School Cook Book*.[15]

CONTINUITIES AND DISCONTINUITIES

At the beginning of the twentieth century, the notion of soul food had not been invented. No equation existed between African American identity and any particular cuisine. Food habits among blacks ranged from the hog-and-hominy traditions of the rural South to the middle-class tastes of the Institute for Colored Youth, where the popularity of beef outranked pork and an appetite for wheat always surpassed a palate for corn.

From the standpoint of culinary tastes and preferences, there was but one obvious thread common to African American culture. The sweet potato had a home everywhere. More than bacon or cornbread, sweet potato occupied an important place in folks' diets from the cotton lands of the Black Belt to the slums of Philadelphia. This was obscured somewhat by its seasonality. From an annual perspective, for instance, sweet potato appeared to be a secondary item in the Tuskegee diet (see table 3.1). When autumn and winter rolled around, however, it stood out as part of the diet's primary core. As such, the sweet potato was fried, boiled, or roasted. It might be baked directly in fire-place ashes or in an oven. Sweet potatoes served as an ingredient in biscuits, breads, muffins, pies, soufflés, and stews. They were baked with pork and apples and sometimes twice baked with brown sugar, raisins, and spices. At the Institute for Colored Youth, the sweet potato often arrived at the table mixed with egg, flour, and baking powder; later, it was fried and served as a puff. It was a dining-hall regular in whatever guise.

In Philadelphia and Washington, where researchers looked at black and white families in identical circumstances, the sweet potato proved to be dis-tinctive. Immigrants from Europe were likely unfamiliar with it; other whites seemed to ignore it. Nationwide, sweet potatoes appeared in about 25 percent of the dietaries gathered during the Atwater era. However, they showed up in nearly 50 percent of the dietaries recorded among African Americans.

Sweet potatoes were a favorite of the nineteenth-century South.[16] However, we cannot assume that the fondness of northern blacks for the sweet potato represented southern heritage. Bacon, a cultural universal among African Americans in the South, counted as a secondary commodity among poor blacks in Philadelphia and Washington. There, bacon was more popular among certain whites, especially English and Irish immigrants, than it was among African Americans. Other southern standbys, including ham, chicken, cornmeal, and hominy, occupied the periphery of the African American diet in Philadelphia and Washington. Pork sausage, rice, beans, and cabbage rated as core items, but these same items were just as popular among whites.

Today we think of all of these foods as important components of the soul food tradition. As such, they represent southern roots and the Afri-can American ancestral experience. A century ago, however, most of these foods were far from prominent on African American tables, even in the rural South. Beans, for example, were all but absent from the typical diets of Tuskegee or Franklin Country. Dried peas and rice were rarely encountered. The Tuskegee series lists cowpeas twice and rice three times. Just one of the dozen families visited in the Dismal Swamp ate peas. None used rice. Leafy

RECIPE 3.2

SWEET POTATO PUFFS

Modern recipes for sweet potato puffs generally call for mashed sweet potatoes combined with milk, butter, eggs, sugar, and other ingredients. The mix gets baked in a casserole or on a cookie sheet.

Fannie Farmer developed a prototype for puffs of this sort, referring to them as "sweet potato balls" or "sweet potato croquettes." Farmer, an accomplished cook who operated a boarding house out of her mother's kitchen, enrolled in the Boston School of Cooking in 1887. She was nominated as the school's principal in 1891. Her most famous work, *The Boston Cooking-School Cook Book*, introduced standardized measures to the kitchen and remains in print to this day.[1]

Ingredients for Fannie Farmer's sweet potato croquettes consisted of two cups of hot, riced sweet potatoes; three tablespoons of butter; a half tablespoon of salt; a few grains of cayenne pepper; the yolk of one egg; and two tablespoons of sherry wine. Farmer instructed readers to cook the potatoes, force them through a ricer, and then add the butter, salt, cayenne pepper, egg yolk, and sherry. The next step was to beat this mixture until very light and shape it into little flat cakes or small spheres. Dip these into crumbs, then into egg, then crumbs again, and finally fry in deep fat. Add more wine to the sweet potato batter should it become too dry.[2]

NOTES

1. Fannie Merritt Farmer, *Boston Cooking-School Cook Book* (Boston: Little, Brown, 1896); "Fannie Farmer," *Wikipedia*, http://en.wikipedia.org/w/index.php?title=Fannie_Farmer&oldid=632145462.

2. Fannie Merritt Farmer, *What to Have for Dinner, Containing Menus with the Recipes Necessary for Their Preparation* (New York: Dodge, 1905).

greens such as collards and mustard, basic to the soul food tradition, were found in just five Tuskegee homes.

Some meats regarded as traditional also made rare appearances. Ham was peripheral to the typical diets of African American households in eastern Virginia and entirely absent from Tuskegee. Chicken showed up in three of the Virginia dietaries and just twice in Tuskegee. The Tuskegee fieldworkers did not see pork sausage at all. The Virginia studies cited it only three times.

Location and season, of course, can be blamed for some these absences. In Franklin County, for instance, the dietaries contained no evidence of anyone eating rice and beans. However, given greater access to markets, rice and beans became mealtime regulars, as exemplified by the typical diet in Elizabeth City–Hampton, where rice qualified as a core item and beans numbered as important peripherals. Conversely, the sweet potato remained a staple in Franklin County even in the spring, but it was missing at that time of the year from menus in the Hampton area. Chicken, absent from Tuskegee households during the cold months, became a peripheral part of the diet in the spring. Fresh pork appeared in 25 percent of Tuskegee's households in the winter, but it went entirely missing in the spring.

While some traditional foods actually may never have been central to African American diets, others lost popularity, moving from isolated, rural settings toward increasingly metropolitan environments. Such was the case with bacon, salt pork, and cornbread. For example, families in Franklin County ate salt sides and belly bacon but almost no beef. Around Hampton, a more commercial area, salt sides remained at the center of the typical diet, but corned beef and other types of cured beef were also popular. Fresh beef and pork, often reduced to sausage, bumped bacon to the secondary core in Philadelphia and Washington and pushed salt pork to the periphery of the typical diet. Finally, at Cheyney we see pork in any form other than ham served only sporadically.

The diminished importance of cornmeal and bacon products in urban and more cosmopolitan settings was largely an economic matter. Cornmeal in eastern Virginia cost families a mere half-cent per kilogram, but in Philadelphia customers paid twice as much. Consequently, Italian immigrants, noted for the inflexibility of their eating habits (see chapter 4), used it more than blacks did. Bacon in rural eastern Virginia could be had for as little as a penny per kilogram. A kilo of salt pork cost about four cents. The price for

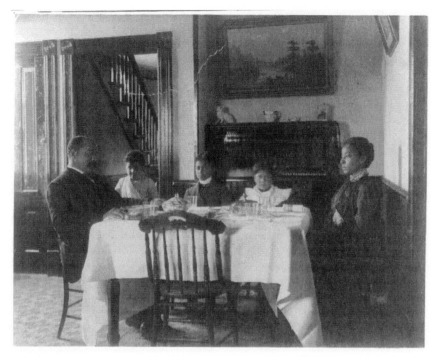

PHOTO 3.3
"Hampton Institute, Va.—a Graduate (Dining) at Home" (c. 1895). The eating habits of the rural South had little influence on diet and nutrition among well-educated blacks and those residing in northern cities. (Photograph by Frances Benjamin Johnston. Courtesy of the Johnston Collection [LC-USZ62-38150], U.S. Library of Congress, Prints and Photographs Division.)

both of these items increased to five cents in Hampton and Philadelphia. At that price, a person could buy fresh pork chops and shoulders. Beef rounds and chuck sold for only a penny or two more. Besides that, spoilage was not the big problem in the cities that it was in rural areas. Nearby shops in the city sold fresh meat in small quantities.

NUTRITIONAL SUPERIORITY OF METROPOLITAN DIETS

Blacks in metropolitan areas were generally better nourished than their rural counterparts. This is evident from the average nutritional values presented in table 3.3. Here the values for Tuskegee represent the diets of tenant farmers and plantation laborers only, and they pertain exclusively to the spring. This renders them directly comparable to the statistics for eastern

Table 3.3.   Average Nutritional Values, Various African American Diets, 1895–1906

PEOPLE & PLACES	Animal CHO (g/m/d)	Animal Protein (g/m/d)	% Energy Animal Fat	% Energy Animal Products	% Food Budget Animal	
Students[1] (fall)	36	79	32	n. d.	n. d.	
Philadelphia—Washington (winter)	17	59	34	44	59	
Elizabeth City—Hampton (spring)	14	57	32	41	61	
Franklin County (spring)	9	54	35	43	59	
Tuskegee (spring)	11	23	33	38	55	
PEOPLE & PLACES	Vegetable CHO (g/m/d)	Total Protein (g/m/d)	Total Fat (g/m/d)	Total Energy (Cal/m/d)	Variety (foods / week) Avg	Variety (foods / week) Max
Students (fall)	378	112	118	3245	22	n. a.
Philadelphia—Washington (winter)	357	107	121	3001	20	30
Elizabeth City—Hampton (spring)	447	110	151	3751	17	27
Franklin County (spring)	445	111	165	3735	4	8
Tuskegee (spring)	499	73	161	3882	4	5

1. per person per day

Virginia. For Philadelphia, all of the dietaries were collected during the winter. The averages for Cheyney apply to fall. Note, however, that in spite of these seasonal differences, and no matter that one set of averages came from urban welfare recipients and the other from an educated elite, the Cheyney and Philadelphia values align closely with one another. Furthermore, their diets rank higher in protein and are more varied in composition than their less metropolitan counterparts.

The Food and Agriculture Organization (FAO) and World Health Organization (WHO) take 0.75 grams of high-quality protein per kilogram of body weight as the world standard for a safe daily allowance.[17] By their yardstick, the protein contents of the diets represented in the table range from marginal or worse at Tuskegee to very generous at the Institute for Colored Youth. Tuskegee's problem was protein quality. The FAO/WHO recommendation, which amounts to 51 g/m/d for an Atwater man-unit, assumes protein sources such as meat, fish, eggs, and milk. The table shows that the Tuskegee diet provided an average of only twenty-three grams of protein per man per day from these types of food. To make matters worse, the table refers to what was probably the highpoint of the year in terms of protein supply (see chapter 4). Franklin County residents did considerably better, owing in part to the ecological complexity of their wetlands and its fish and game resources. The average intake of protein from animal sources in Elizabeth City County and Hampton was slightly higher than Franklin County's, and in Philadelphia the intake was higher still. Nevertheless, the intake of animal protein in all of these communities was generally inferior to averages for poor whites (see chapter 4). This was not true of total protein intakes, however. From Franklin County to Philadelphia, the total protein content of diets was comparable, on average, to white Americans, including salaried professionals (see chapter 4). Similarly, the total protein value of meals served at the Institute for Colored Youth averaged about the same as that of white students (see chapter 6).

Indeed, if one takes averages at the Institute for Colored Youth as generally indicative of nutrition among comfortably situated blacks, it would appear there was nothing particularly distinctive about African American nutrition at the metropolitan end of the continuum. The cooks at Cheyney prepared meals along standard lines. The school's menu for the first fifteen days of October shows that the dining hall regularly met modern USDA minimum serving recommendations in the "meat," "dairy," and "vegetable" categories. In the area of "fruits," students received the prescribed minimum of two servings about every other day, but every day there was at least one fruit on the table. A minimum of three different items from the "bread, cereal, rice, and pasta" group were offered daily. An extra slice or two of bread and second helpings would have provided the six servings recommended for this category. The biggest problem, perhaps, was the two to five daily servings of "fats, oils and sweets," foods the USDA advised people to "use sparingly." Total fat intake at Cheyney was about the same as that recorded among African Americans living in Philadelphia and Washington, but it averaged considerably less than the corresponding figures for blacks in Alabama and eastern Virginia. This stands to reason in light of the total energy intakes documented in those places (see table 3.3). The resident farmers and their families needed considerably more energy than student boarders and found a cheap source in animal fat.

Oddly, the data presented in table 3.3 do not indicate the different penchants for animal products associated with the nutrition transition. In the previous chapter, urban dwellers and students, constituents of economically developed areas, consumed more meat products than their neighbors in the mountains. Here, judging from the proportion of energy drawn from animal fat, the students at the Institute for Colored Youth, and, for that matter, the poor families of Philadelphia and Washington, appear to have been no more inclined toward foods derived from animals than the residents of Tuskegee or Franklin County. This can be explained by the fact that neither Tuskegee nor Franklin County were awaiting development. Both had been enmeshed in the industrial world for more than a century. Franklin County had "regressed." Following emancipation and the collapse of the "factory-in-field" regime of the slave plantation, folks found refuge in the Dismal Swamp, where they lived as a kind of subsistence-oriented quasi-peasantry. Around Tuskegee, that was never an option. Farmers all across the Black Belt had to pin their hopes on cash crops while sustaining themselves on credit and mostly store-bought foods. Thus, communities that on the surface seemed out of the economic mainstream were actually closely attuned to it.

This involvement expressed itself in social institutions such as going to shop on Saturday mornings. This exercise was as ritualistic as it was practical. From midmorning on, tenants and laborers converged on towns and crossroad stores, ostensibly to pick up a few supplies.[18] The actual purchases might have taken one person a short time to accomplish. Nonetheless, entire families made the trip, and everyone spent half of the day standing about the storefronts smoking and conversing. The scene on Sunday shifted from the "shopping center" to the church or, as Washington put it, to "some big meeting."[19] This gathering ideally was to be followed in the afternoon by a substantial dinner, but as far as the rest of the week was concerned, there was little of the daily bread-breaking that supposedly brings families together. Sitting down at the table to eat a meal was an awkward experience because family members usually ate alone and often on the go.[20] Mealtimes on workdays proceeded as if straight out of a manufacturing setting. The man of the house would take his breakfast in hand and be out the door on his way to his field, eating his bacon and cornbread as he went. His wife regularly took her meal alone, right from the frying pan. The children too young to help in the fields ate in snatches while amusing themselves outside in the yard.

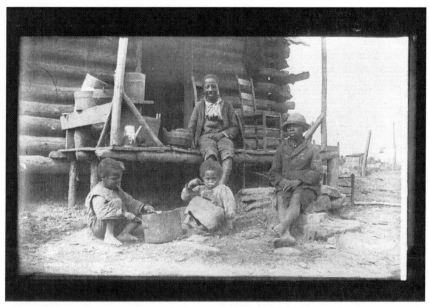

PHOTO 3.4
"Living Easy" (c. 1895). Children too young to work in the fields usually ate outside in the yard. (Courtesy of the Detroit Publishing Company Photograph Collection [LC-DIG-det-4a27228], U.S. Library of Congress, Prints and Photographs Division.)

The only thing genuinely "folk" about the Tuskegee diet was its plainness and simplicity. During the spring, no ordinary cotton farmer used more than five different commodities per week (see table 3.3). For Franklin County's families, there was greater geographic potential for diversity, but for many it went unrealized. Thus, as table 3.3 indicates, one household used eight food items per week. Others consumed just two or three. Elizabeth City–Hampton residents, fully engaged with metropolitan markets, enjoyed far greater variety with a weekly average of seventeen distinct foods. The average came to twenty-two items per week for families living in town. But, surprisingly, welfare clients in Philadelphia did even better (see table 3.3). For that matter, the two nearly destitute Washington, DC, families studied by Foreman purchased an average of thirteen different foods per week, in effect enjoying a much greater variety of foods than the farmers that the OES surveyed in the South. Comparing average food expenditures among all of the groups for which we have data suggests that when African Americans had more money to spend on food, they opted to diversify their diets rather than simply to eat more of the same.

Here it is important to stress that the issue was not migration. At this point in American history, blacks did not regularly relocate from the South to the North or move from rural to urban locations. Nonetheless, some have interpreted the lack of interest in pork, cornbread, and other icons of southern cuisine among urban blacks prior to World War I as a kind of betrayal of African American culture. Tracy Poe, for instance, has portrayed the origins of soul food as a matter of African Americans no longer being willing to "bend down to anyone" but just being themselves.[21] According to Poe, black Chicagoans prior to the Great Migration held fast to the integrationist philosophy of Booker Washington and aspired to respectable, middle-class white values. Consequently, they emulated Euro-American foodways, and they looked down on southern blacks and their tastes as backward.

Unfortunately, Richards and Shapleigh offered no information about how the families they sampled felt about southern cooking, nor do we know how the men and women attending the Institute for Colored Youth might react to the typical foods of the Black Belt. Nevertheless, there are data to suggest that cost and convenience were of concern. Folks in the city were not about to eat in a hog-and-hominy tradition when lean meat could be had for about the same price as pork fat and cornmeal was more expensive than wheat flour. The stage for the eventual success of southern-style food in the urban North would be set soon enough by the Great Migration and the arrival of masses of people anxious for a taste of home. Its christening as "soul food" awaited the arrival of the late 1950s and newfound commercial and political values attached to ethnic identity. By this time, the infrastructure would be fully in place to eat like an Alabama cotton farmer who somehow was able to put the foods of spring, summer, fall, and winter on the table all at once at any time of the year. As a cultural ideal, the soul food tradition never entertains a worry about a winter of unremitting bacon, cornbread, and molasses.

4

Rich and Poor and the Seasonality of Diet

America one hundred years ago had a three-tiered class system that was somewhat more clearly delineated than today's. At the top, a wealthy upper class owned and directed the nation's most profitable and most powerful organizations. Members of the middle class, whose incomes ranged from copious to barely comfortable, managed and staffed these organizations. They also owned a variety of lesser properties and administered the nation's educational and cultural institutions. Small farmers and a heterogeneous working class populated the lower echelons of society. Skilled and semiskilled mechanics and tradesmen made up about 15 percent of the working class. They generally earned sufficient income to eat well, dress respectably, and buy a home. Members of the working class whose labors did not demand special skills netted just enough to eat, pay rent, and meet other basic needs. When an unskilled laborer lost his job or fell ill, his family fell into penury within a matter of weeks. An estimated 20 percent of the working class existed in this condition.

This chapter compares patterns of food consumption across class lines. It pays particular attention to the middle class and the working-class poor. Food histories, most notably Harvey Levenstein's *Revolution at the Table*, have covered this same ground.[1] However, sparse information about lower-class eating habits has proved to be a big stumbling block, resulting in dim appreciation of how poverty affected nutrition.[2]

The Atwater-era dietaries shed considerable light on the issue. They confirm that members of the middle class had more to eat than common laborers, and they bear out that the foods purchased by the middle class were generally of higher quality and more costly than those bought by members of the working class. But if these inequities almost go without saying, there remains much to learn about the nutritional consequences of seasonality. In this regard, a careful inspection of dietaries collected from both middle-class and working-class families reveals remarkable annual fluctuations in nutrition and the existence of veritable "hungry months," especially among subjects of modest means.[3] This helps explain the stunted growth that affected members of the American working class throughout the Gilded Age and well into the twentieth century.

UPPER- AND MIDDLE-CLASS DIETS

The food habits of the upper echelon of American society received a great deal of publicity during the Gilded Age. People read regularly about high society's magnificent dinner parties featuring dishes prepared by French chefs. The newspapers told of waiters setting tables with enormous amounts of food, and by all accounts rich celebrities and other wealthy diners tucked it away enthusiastically. No one imagined it shameful to look overstuffed.[4] After-dinner photographs showed brandy and cigars and men's bellies protruding from their waistcoats. Women's fashion favored ample bosoms, sturdy hips, and strapping buttocks, all testifying to a healthy appetite for rich cuisine. There is no doubting Levenstein's contention that holding one's own at a splendidly appointed table was, for the upper crust, an important validation of status.[5]

Early nutritionists did not document upper-class nutrition directly. The rich, after all, were not supposed to be the problem. Researchers did pay attention to the middle class, but at first this was primarily a matter of expediency—a matter of chemists measuring their own food intakes and monitoring the consumption of colleagues because it was the cheapest, easiest way for scientists studying food and nutrition to collect data. Later on, a set of studies carried out in Chicago in 1895, featuring the families of a suburban school superintendent and two college professors, was deliberately embarked on in order to put the diets of poor immigrants in comparative perspective.[6] While no direct reference was made to the concept of economic class as such, the term "professional" was used as a kind of euphemism for middle-class status. First-generation nutritionists also pointed to middle-class status in an oblique way by noting the presence of household servants or by characterizing a family's economic circumstances as "comfortable." These indicators appeared in the context of thirteen dietaries or roughly 3 percent of the entire corpus of native-born household dietaries produced during the Atwater era.[7]

Table 4.1 outlines a typical diet from late fall through winter based on food consumption data gleaned from six middle-class households situated in vari-

Table 4.1. Typical Fall–Winter Diet, Middle-Class Households, Northeastern and Midwestern States, 1895–1897

	Meat and Dairy	Grains and Dried Legumes	Fats, Oils, Sugars, and Starches	Roots and Tubers	Other Vegetables	Fruits and Misc.
Primary Core	fresh beef[1] fresh pork[2] egg milk cheese[3]	wheat flour cornmeal oatmeal[4] rice wheat bread crackers[5]	lard butter sugar	potato		apple orange
Secondary Core	dried beef[6] veal[7] lamb, mutton[8] bacon, salt pork ham chicken fresh fish[9] oysters	barley cake[10] macaroni bean[8]	honey maple syrup molasses starch[11] tapioca	onion sweet potato	cabbage lettuce canned corn	tomato banana dried peach prunes cranberry canned fruit[12]
Periphery	beef kidney beef liver pork sausage clams cream	buckwheat cracked wheat Graham flour rye flour hominy brown bread rolls	brown sugar tapioca	parsnip radish turnip peanuts	soup greens prunella[13] canned peas pickles	dates grapes preserves[14]

1. diverse cuts, including rib roast, and a variety of steaks
2. variety of cuts
3. Swiss and other unspecified varieties
4. and rolled oats
5. including cream, Graham, milk, oyster, soda, and unspecified varieties
6. including smoked beef
7. chops and cutlets
8. variety of cuts, including chops
9. California salmon and lake trout
10. fig cake and unspecified types
11. types not specified
12. including cherries and plums
13. a salad and pot herb
14. including tomato

ous parts of the Northeast and Midwest, including Lafayette, Indiana; New York City; Pittsburgh; Storrs, Connecticut; and Urbana, Illinois.[8] The table shows a small number of invariably present commodities, including fresh beef, lard, eggs, butter, milk, cheese, wheat flour, granulated sugar, and potatoes. These and most of the other foods listed were needed to cook the classic American dishes of the era.

The idea that there was a standard set of all-American dishes—a national cuisine, if you will—was new. Ellen Richards, a founder of the home economics movement in the United States, helped develop and promote the concept. She intended it as an alternative to European cooking traditions and as a way to counteract the allegedly extravagant eating habits of immigrants.[9] Inspired by rural New England cooking, all-American menus typically featured forced and pressed meats, fresh fish, clams, cracked wheat, corn and oatmeal mush, brown bread, baked beans, corn chowder, boiled hominy, succotash, and Indian pudding (see recipe 4.1).[10] Middle-class American cookbooks added white sauces and composed salads, attempting to enliven what was otherwise a rather plain collection of dishes.[11]

Although the American middle class contented itself with simple cookery, its diet was exceedingly varied. Even in the midst of winter, middle-class families experienced none of the monotony described in previous chapters. For core grains, table 4.1 lists not only wheat but also corn, rice, oats, and barley. Buckwheat qualified as a peripheral food and was consumed mostly in the winter. The day of the buckwheat pancake, the classic nineteenth-century American breakfast food, was in decline. Nonetheless, maple syrup, the standard pancake topping, was a core item. Spring inventories listed commercial breakfast cereals, including the Wheatlet and Wheatina brand names. These were newcomers to the table; yet they ranked as secondary core foods. Macaroni, a long-standing favorite of the upper class, was also part of the secondary core. Americans regarded macaroni as a luxury food as late as 1886. Soon afterward, it became more affordable and popular thanks to the enterprise of Italian immigrants.[12]

The evident liking for commercially baked bread and cakes indicated in table 4.1 might come as a surprise. Americans at this point in history were supposed to have remained strongly attached to home baking. According to food historian Richard Hooker, they harbored lingering suspicions about whether baker's bread was clean and wholesome.[13] But seeing as it showed up in close

INDIAN PUDDINGS

The name "Indian pudding" alludes to the Native American origin of corn, the pudding's principal ingredient. Indian pudding originated as an Americanized version of hasty pudding, a British mainstay made of wheat flour cooked in boiling milk or water to the point of turning into a thick batter.[1] American colonists substituted cornmeal for wheat, which they lacked, and insisted on milk, of which they had plenty. They added to the pudding locally produced sweeteners, such as molasses or maple syrup, perhaps some cinnamon or ginger, and maybe one or two other refinements. The batter, no matter what was added, could be boiled or baked.

Both versions diminished in popularity over the years but then resurged following the Civil War, when Thanksgiving Day became a federal holiday. Influential journalists advocated a Thanksgiving celebration modeled after New England tradition, which, among other things, meant a big dinner featuring North American species. Indian pudding fit right in and became a popular component of the feast. Within a few years, its appeal expanded to the point of making it a cold-weather standby on the dinner tables of the middle class.[2]

Recipes for boiled and baked Indian puddings could be found in every cookbook published during the Gilded Age, including the very popular *Buckeye Cookery, and Practical Housekeeping: Compiled from Original Recipes*.[3] It first appeared 1876 as a charity cookbook put together by the women of the First Congregational Church of Marysville, Ohio. Estelle Woods Wilcox, editor of the original collection, purchased the copyright. She and her husband then proceeded to publish subsequent editions.[4]

The Wilcoxes attributed their recipe for "plain boiled Indian pudding" to Mrs. L. S. W.[5] Her recipe called for one and a half pints of Indian meal (cornmeal), a half pint of boiling water, four tablespoons of Graham flour, one pint of milk (either soured or mixed with a little salt), two tablespoons of molasses, a half teaspoon of ginger, salt, one level teaspoon of baking soda, and two tablespoons of chopped suet (optional for a lighter, more tender pudding). Preparation required scalding the cornmeal in the boiling water as a first step. The pot was then removed from

(*continued*)

the heat, and the Graham flour, milk, molasses, ginger, soda, and a little salt were added to it. The suet, if so desired, needed to be added at this point as well. One then placed the mixture into a well-greased, two-quart pudding boiler—essentially a double boiler—leaving room for the pudding to swell. Boiling time was three to four hours. Optionally, the mixture could be tied into a pudding cloth—again, leaving room to swell—and boiled or steamed for three to four hours.

Mrs. Carrier received credit for *Buckeye Cookery*'s "bake Indian pudding."[6] Her recipe required one quart of milk, one ounce of butter, four well-beaten eggs, one cup of cornmeal, a half pound of raisins, and a quarter pound of sugar. To start with, the milk was scalded with the cornmeal and stirred as the milk boiled. Once the cornmeal was blended into the milk, the pot was removed from the burner and allowed to stand until "blood warm." At that point, one stirred in the remaining ingredients and baked for one and a half hours. The recipe directed serving the pudding hot, covered with sauce. Mrs. A. E. Brand, author of yet another *Buckeye Cookery* recipe for Indian pudding, suggested a sauce made of drawn butter, wine, and nutmeg.[7] Other cookbooks suggested brandy hard sauce, caramel sauce, and maple syrup.

NOTES

1. "Hasty Pudding," *Wikipedia*, http://en.wikipedia.org/w/index. php?title=Hasty_pudding&oldid=639492437.

2. Ibid.

3. Estelle Woods Wilcox, *Buckeye Cookery, and Practical Housekeeping: Compiled from Original Recipes* (Marysville, OH: Buckeye, 1877).

4. Anne-Marie Rachman, "*Buckeye Cookery*," *Feeding America: The Historic American Cookbook Project*, Digital and Multimedia Center, Michigan State University Libraries, http://digital.lib.msu.edu/projects/cookbooks/html/books/book_33.cfm.

5. Wilcox, *Buckeye Cookery*, 202.

6. Ibid.

7. Ibid., 201.

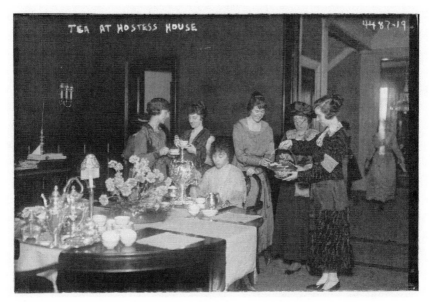

PHOTO 4.1
"Tea at Hostess House" (no date). Tea time was an important institution among the upper classes. Women visited daily over light refreshments and talked about events in their community. (Photograph by Bain News Service. Courtesy of the George Grantham Bain Collection [LC-DIG-ggbain-26171], U.S. Library of Congress, Prints and Photographs Division.)

to half of the middle-class dietaries collected by first-generation nutritionists, attitudes must have been changing. Commercially baked crackers or biscuits of various sorts (cream crackers, milk crackers, oyster crackers, Graham crackers, etc.), which by this time were sold in sanitary packages, had an even more ubiquitous presence in middle-class homes than store-bought bread.

Members of the middle class partook of as much variety in the domain of animal products as they did in the sphere of grains. The beef rounds, rib roasts, shoulder cuts, and various steaks listed in table 4.1 amounted to staples. Homemakers fried streaks, cut thin, for both breakfast and dinner and served them with a pan gravy. The more discriminating insisted on named cuts, such as porterhouse or sirloin, preferably dished up with grilled onions, mushrooms, or tomatoes. More than any other dish, patrons of New York restaurants called for roast beef, cooked rare.[14] As shown in the table, people in comfortable circumstances had a taste for dried and smoked beef as well. Fresh pork had a primary place in the diet during the cold-weather months, but as temperatures warmed, veal, bacon, ham, and fresh fish moved up from the secondary core to replace it.

Table 4.1 shows the middle class commanding a large assortment of vegetables and fruits. Kitchens stocked the usual winter roots, supplemented with a variety of canned species. Cabbage and lettuce kept a green component in the core diet throughout the cold-weather months. Farmers in the South had begun growing salad greens and other vegetables for northern markets soon after the Civil War. By 1889, northern cities were receiving winter shipments of cauliflower, cucumber, eggplant, radish, spinach, and onions.[15] Tomatoes came from the South, as well as from local hothouses. By the turn of the century, California shipped oranges, raisins, table grapes, apples, peaches, pears, plums, apricots, figs, and olives.[16] About the same time, oranges and bananas became popular alternatives to winter apples. Steamships made bananas available to consumers on the East Coast for most of the year.[17] Interior markets were not so well supplied. Still, in middle-class dietaries logged during the spring months, bananas appeared right alongside strawberries, the locally grown seasonal fruit.

The precise manner in which middle-class consumers ate fruits and vegetables was immaterial in the view of early nutritionists. Menus and recipes did not concern them. Still, surviving bills of fare from noncommercial venues, mostly institutions of higher learning, help complete the picture. These are relevant because students boarding at colleges and universities came, for the most part, from well-off middle- and upper-class backgrounds, and many schools were keen on offering them homelike accommodations. At the University of Chicago, for example, administrators decided in 1894 to experiment with menus modeled on the home.[18] The idea was to foster scholastic success by providing well-balanced meals composed of a limited variety of foods prepared in the best possible manner. The foods themselves were to be relatively low cost, but they were to be expertly made and attractively served. The study involved three adjoining residence halls—Kelly, Beecher, and Nancy Foster—each providing room and board for forty female undergraduates. The residences contained separate dining rooms, but the bulk of the cooking took place in Kelly Hall because of its central location. There the university installed equipment recently used in the famous Rumford Kitchen, a working exhibition of scientific cookery and nutrition information, which had been installed the year before on the grounds of the nearby Chicago World's Columbian Exposition.

BOILED LEG OF LAMB IN CAPER SAUCE

Maria Parloa, better known as Miss Parloa, has been hailed as America's first celebrity cook.[1] She burst onto the scene in the early 1870s as a cookbook author and lecturer in the Boston area. As her career progressed, she became a recognized expert in domestic science, a noted lecturer at the Boston Cooking School, founder of her own cooking schools, food editor of *Good Housekeeping* magazine, and spokeswoman for several big food companies.[2] Her best-selling cookbook, *Miss Parloa's New Cook Book*, first appeared in 1880 and went through ten editions.[3] It contained a recipe for boiled leg of lamb a la Francaise.

Few people would think of boiling a leg of lamb these days.[4] Now, simply roasting one is generally considered all that is necessary to produce a delicious centerpiece for dinner. Miss Parloa's recipe is truly Gilded Age, an apt representation of the taste of the privileged classes for elaborate dishes. Her instructions—considered a model of clarity—are presented here in her own words.[5]

Put a leg of lamb, weighing about eight pounds, in as small a kettle as will hold it. Put in a muslin bag one onion, one small white turnip, a few green celery leaves, three sprigs each of sweet marjoram and summer savory, four cloves and twelve allspice. Tie the bag and place it in the kettle with the lamb; then pour on two quarts of boiling water. Let this come to a boil, and then skim carefully. Now add four heaping table-spoonfuls of flour, which has been mixed with one cupful of cold water, two table-spoonfuls of salt and a speck of cayenne. Cover tight, and set back where it will just simmer for four hours. In the meantime make a pint and a half of veal or mutton force-meat, which make into little balls and fry brown. Boil six eggs hard. At the end of four hours take up the lamb. Skim all the fat off of the gravy and take out the bag of seasoning. Now put the kettle where the contents will boil rapidly for ten minutes. Put three table-spoonfuls of butter in the frying-pan, and when hot, stir in two of flour; cook until a dark brown, but not burned, and stir into the gravy.

(*continued*)

Taste to see if seasoned enough. Have the whites and yolks of the hard-boiled eggs chopped separately. Pour the gravy over the lamb; then garnish with the chopped eggs, making a hill of the whites, and capping it with part of the yolks. Sprinkle the remainder of the yolks over the lamb. Place the meat balls in groups around the dish. Garnish with parsley, and serve.[6]

To serve the leg of lamb in caper sauce, omit preparing the gravy and garnishes as described above and instead make Miss Parloa's favorite caper sauce. It required two tablespoons of flour, a half cup of butter, one pint of boiling water, one tablespoon of lemon juice, two tablespoons of capers, and one tablespoon of essence of anchovy (perhaps anchovy paste or juice). The recipe began with working the butter and flour together until creamy and then gradually adding the boiling water. This liquid was then returned to a boil and immediately removed from the stove. The lemon juice, capers, and essence of anchovy were stirred in just before serving.[7]

NOTES

1. "Maria Parloa," *Wikipedia*, http://en.wikipedia.org/w/index.php?title=Maria_Parloa&oldid=611937608.

2. Ibid.

3. Maria Parloa, *Miss Parloa's New Cookbook: A Guide to Marketing and Cooking* (New York: C. T. Dillingham, 1882), first published 1880 by Estes and Lauriat.

4. Even in Parloa's time, the more common dish was boiled mutton, often accompanied by caper sauce.

5. Anne-Marie Rachman, "Miss Parloa: Maria Parloa (September 25, 1843–August 21, 1909)," *Feeding America: The Historic American Cookbook Project*, Digital and Multimedia Center, Michigan State University Libraries, http://digital.lib.msu.edu/projects/cookbooks/html/authors/author_parloa.html.

6. Parloa, *Miss Parloa's New Cookbook*, 138–39.

7. Ibid., 227–28.

A report on the university's project itemized detailed menus for three consecutive weeks, beginning March 1.[19] On that day, breakfast consisted of grapefruit, farinose,[20] creamed codfish, and baked potatoes. As always, butter, milk, cream, sugar, bread, and rolls were also on the table, and the students had a choice of coffee, tea, or cocoa to drink. An assortment of meats, cold ham, sausages, and corned beef, was served for lunch, accompanied by creamed potatoes and peaches. Dinner began with beef soup and a lettuce salad. Boiled lamb in caper sauce (see recipe 4.2), mashed potatoes, and canned corn followed. Delicate pudding was served for dessert.[21]

Ellen Richards, who consulted on the project, and university official Marion Talbot calculated the average numbers of macronutrients consumed over the course of the experiment.[22] Average intakes per coed amounted to 108 g/d of protein, 103 g/d of fat, and 387 g/d of carbohydrates with a total fuel value of 2,953 Cal/d. These figures were not out of line with those derived from the study of the three middle-class, Chicago-area families referred to at the beginning of this section.[23]

WHAT MEMBERS OF THE WORKING CLASS ATE

As Levenstein's *Revolution at the Table* progresses down the social ladder and approaches the topic of "how the other half live," his literary sources peter out.[24] Rich descriptions give way to vague characterizations. The narrative becomes especially thin when it tackles the matter of what the urban poor ate and how they fared nutritionally.

This picture can be fleshed out thanks to three major research projects and the considerable amount of information that they produced. Ellen Richards and Amelia Shapleigh directed the first of these undertakings in Chicago in 1893.[25] W. O. Atwater organized a second in New York City beginning in 1895.[26] Several years later, S. E. Forman's *Conditions of Living among the Poor* appeared.[27] It reported the results of a large-scale budgetary and standard-of-living inquiry conducted in Washington, DC. It stands out today as our only systematically constructed record of food consumption for the urban South prior to the Great Depression.

On Chicago's West Side

Richards and Shapleigh's study, conducted during the spring of 1893, generated a total of thirty-one dietaries. The investigators worked out of Hull

House, Chicago's most prominent settlement agency, and studied households located in its immediate vicinity.[28] This crowded Near West Side neighborhood hosted many thousands of immigrants from Europe, whose eating habits come up for consideration in the next chapter. Of concern here are the native-born, working-class residents of the area as represented by a subset of thirteen households that agreed to take part in the study.[29] These families typified the skilled and semi-skilled elements of the working class. Most of the adult women belonged to the Women's Club at Hull House, and most of their families enjoyed "good incomes." The children in one case appeared underfed, but generally speaking the youngsters looked remarkably healthy.

In some respects, the typical diet of these families differed substantially from the diets of the middle and upper classes. Unlike the latter, whose members often ate beef in the form of rib roast and short loin steaks, this sector of the working class dined mainly on shoulder and rump roasts and inexpensive steaks (round and sirloin). Furthermore, families did not usually eat the lamb or chicken consumed by middle-class householders, nor did they regularly sit down to turkey like the women boarding at the University of Chicago. The wage earners near Hull House typically favored fresh pork and mutton. These meats constituted core foods among the middle class as well, but they were not central to the typical diet of the upper class.

White sugar and butter were common to the tables of all classes. However, in middle- and upper-class homes researchers were more apt to find a variety of other sweeteners, including brown sugar, honey, maple syrup, and molasses. Alternatives to butter were more likely to be encountered among the families of laborers. Their cupboards often contained butterine, a butter substitute containing 40 percent dairy fat. Butterine consisted of butter, margarine, and lard, with annatto and turmeric added for coloring. Other popular butter substitutes used by families on tight budgets were margarine and cottolene. The margarine of the late nineteenth century consisted of a mixture of beef fat, milk, salt, and artificial coloring agents. Cottolene was a compound of cottonseed oil and oleostearin from beef fat. Around 1900, an estimated 6 percent of all households in the United States used one or more of these ersatz butters.[30]

Around Rundown Parts of Washington, DC

S. E. Forman's account of household expenditures among the poor of Washington, DC, provides a good starting point for understanding the eat-

ing habits of unskilled workers because of its lucid account of living conditions and domestic economy.[31] The study covered nineteen households. The
seventeen considered here consisted of white families who, like the African
Americans referred to in the previous chapter, lived hand to mouth. If they
did not represent absolutely the neediest people in the city, it was because Forman knew that the totally destitute were incapable of fruitfully collaborating
with him. Consequently, he ventured as far down the scale of fortunes as he
could, stopping just short of where sobriety, honesty, and industry melted into
economic despair and ruined any prospect for careful and honest record keeping. Families at that point still hovered dangerously close to the financial edge.
No more than one month of unemployment, in Forman's estimation, stood
between their current level of poverty and absolute pennilessness.[32]

Forman found his subjects in various parts of the district. Generally
speaking, they occupied rental houses or apartments no larger than three
or four rooms. These were in disrepair and had no running water or other
conveniences. Household size averaged between six and seven members. The
principal wage earner in most cases was male. Several of the men made their
living with a pick and shovel. Two worked as teamsters. One was employed as
a tinner, another as a clerk. Wives earned additional income in two households.
Three women supported families on their own. Gainful employment invariably
involved cleaning, laundering, or sewing. Agreeing to participate in Forman's
research entailed the added work of keeping track of earnings and expenses for
a total of five weeks—three continuous weeks during the summer or early fall
of 1905 and another two weeks the following January or February.

Irrespective of the time of year, food comprised the families' biggest expense. Grocery bills usually amounted to something between 45 and 55 percent of their income. Costs in some instances ran higher, but anything beyond
two-thirds of a family's earnings led to terrible difficulties. Forman illustrated
this with the story of one family that spent, on average, 67 percent of its weekly
income on food and soon found itself unable to meet other needs. This com-
pelled a search for cheaper rooms and a move to the far outskirts of the city.
The new area, as it turned out, had no schools. This left the hapless couple in
the painful position of having sacrificed their children's education in exchange
for being better able to satisfy their demands for food.

Households with exceptionally high food costs usually had a surfeit of
growing boys.[33] Their loud and incessant cries for food wore parents down

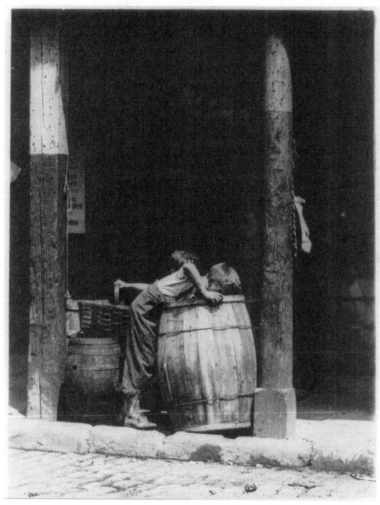

PHOTO 4.2
"This Boy and Brother Were Picking Discarded Fruit out of Barrels in Market near 14th St. N.Y. City . . ." (1910). The boys stole good fruit when they
thought no one was looking. (Photograph by Lewis Wickes Hine. Courtesy of
the records of the National Child Labor Committee [LC-DIG-nclc-04678], U.S.
Library of Congress, Prints and Photographs Division.)

to the point of giving up. Among his subjects, Forman met a couple with six
children literally being eaten out of house and home.[34] The family lived in
three dirty rooms above a grocery store. The father worked, when he could,
at bridge construction to earn twelve dollars a week. One son also worked,
bringing home about a third of that amount. Fifty-five percent of the house-

hold's total income went for food. The family needed eleven dollars a month for rent. It was overdue, and there was no money for much-needed clothing. The couple relieved their situation by sending two sons away to a local industrial school, where they would be fed and clothed at public expense.

Forman did not subscribe to the popular doctrine that the poor needed to be taught how to spend their food dollars wisely. To the contrary, he saw his subjects as astutely rational. If they ate mostly bread, spending as much as 25 percent of their food dollars at the baker's shop, it was because at five cents a loaf there was no better nutritional bargain (except for stale loaves, which were available at four cents or less). The cost of oven fuel alone banished any thought of home-baked bread or rolls. Time was also a consideration. If oatmeal was not on the menu for breakfast, it was not because parents were careless, but rather because harried homemakers in poverty-stricken households could ill afford time in the morning to prepare a hot breakfast.

The core diet of impoverished Washingtonians consisted of thirty-six foods during the summer and early autumn and thirty during the winter. Items from animals in the winter diet typically included eggs, fresh beef, fresh pork, ham (various types, including canned), fresh fish (principally mackerel), bologna, fresh milk, condensed milk, butter, cheese, and lard. This might give the impression of a diet rich in animal-sourced commodities. However, the quantities purchased were generally very small, and these families spent little on meat and dairy compared to the more fortunate. Nonetheless, meats, on average, took about 30 percent of the food budget. Homemakers bought fresh pork mainly as chops, pudding, sausage, and shoulder. Beef purchases most often included liver, unspecified steaks, shoulder, stew meat, and soup bones. Three of Forman's families ate chicken during the late summer and fall. All of them ate fish regardless of the season. Only seven families drank milk daily, and many let weeks go by without buying butter. Still, dairy products were eliminated from the diet entirely only when a breadwinner was unemployed or when some other emergency arose. Families showed a similar reluctance to eliminate meat from the diet.

When push came to shove, the first foods pared from shopping lists were fruits and vegetables other than potatoes. These endured as the backbone of the diet year round. Onions and cabbages normally joined potatoes to form a trinity of primary vegetables. Tomatoes and fresh, sweet corn became part of the core when they were in season. Turnips assumed the status of a secondary mainstay during the cold months. Apples predominated among the fruits during the harvest months, but by January fruits came to the table mainly in the form of preserves. Because people usually spread preserves on bread, Forman referred to them as "butter substitutes."[35]

The Washington budgetaries tell of seasonal shifts in core meat consumption. Lamb, a core item during the summer, failed to appear in winter inventories; beef liver and pork pudding showed up instead. The same with codfish; its place as a core food in the typical warm-weather diet fell to mackerel during the winter months.

Inside the Tenements of New York City

Atwater brought the OES and its nutrition studies to New York City in 1895 with the promise of investigating purchasing patterns, prices, and the accuracy of weights and measures.[36] According to plan, the agency's research would concentrate on blighted neighborhoods where residents allegedly did not receive fair value for money spent on food. By the time the project was finished in 1897, the OES had records of what fifty-eight families had consumed over periods of at least seven days.[37] Twenty-seven of these records pertained to families native to the United States.

Nearly all of the subjects involved depended, to some degree, on charity. Most of them made their homes in squalid tenements near the intersection of Cherry and Catherine streets. A handful lived on the West Side near Forty-Third Street and Eleventh Avenue. People in both places subsisted on little more than the essentials, purchasing small quantities of food from neighborhood shops day by day or even meal by meal. Yet in only three cases was the principal wage earner unemployed at the time of the study. Several of the men worked as common laborers. One found employment as an expressman. Another worked in a foundry. Other occupations included janitor, longshoreman, painter, peddler, and waiter. Women, variously employed as cleaners and launderers, were the principal or sole source of income for seven families.

Atwater's New York project, like his earlier efforts in Alabama and Chicago, depended on local expertise. It came in this instance from the New York Association for the Improvement of the Condition of the Poor and its "district visitors." These social workers were called upon to do the project's legwork and keep track of what Atwater's subjects ate. Isabelle Delaney, a physician, did the bulk of this fieldwork. She had considerable experience serving the Lower East Side both as a missionary and as a medical practitioner. Her facility for understanding the worldview of slum dwellers and making sense of their ideas impressed Atwater. Delaney's sympathies were unreservedly with those in the tenements, and they reciprocated by gamely submitting to her inquiries. Before she and her fellow district visitors were through, they were able to file a substantial collection of information that, taken as a whole, specifies consumption patterns throughout an entire year.[38]

Table 4.2 represents a typical diet. Its contents capture the results of thirteen household inventories conducted from January through late March and indicating what poor, unskilled laborers ate between growing seasons.

Table 4.2. Typical January–March Diet of Poor Working-Class Families, New York City, 1897

	Meat and Dairy	Grains and Dried Legumes	Fats, Oils, Sugars, and Starches	Roots and Tubers	Other Vegetables	Fruits and Misc.
Primary Core	fresh beef[1] corned beef fresh fish[2] egg milk cheese[3]	wheat bread cracker[4] buns[5]	butter sugar	onion potato	cabbage	tomato[6]
Secondary Core	beef tripe[7] boiled ham mutton[8] salt cod canned salmon oyster condensed milk	wheat flour oatmeal barley rye bread roll[9] cake[10] beans peas		carrot turnip radish	soup greens	prune
Periphery	fresh veal lamb pork variety[11] pork sausage chicken	rice muffin	lard molasses corn starch		canned corn catsup	apple

1. diverse cuts
2. herring, smelt, and cod
3. unspecified types
4. mostly soda crackers
5. assorted types
6. fresh and canned
7. pickled
8. diverse cuts
9. various kinds
10. a variety of types
11. includes corned pork, headcheese, and trimmings

Not surprisingly, the table does not list many vegetables and fruits. For Gilded Age Americans in general, and most certainly for the poor, winter's vegetables and fruits were limited to those few items amenable to cold storage, a few canned and dried products, and possibly one or two hothouse (greenhouse) species. Very likely, the greens and some of the tomatoes listed in the typical diet were grown under glass. Canned tomatoes were more common, however. The only other fruit inventoried with some frequency was the prune. In stark contrast, the typical winter diet of the middle class contained seven core fruits, including apples, oranges, and bananas (see table 4.1).

Under the heading of primary core meats, poor New Yorkers consumed both fresh and corned beef, as well as a variety of fresh fish. Secondary core meats included beef tripe, boiled ham, salt cod, and canned salmon. Missing from the core of the typical working-class diet, yet frequently present on middle-class tables, were cuts of fresh lamb, pork, and veal; dried and smoked beef; cured pork, including bacon, ham, and salted pieces; and chicken. Other products not regularly documented among the poor were cornmeal, rice, and macaroni. When it came to baked goods, they used half as many grains and grain varieties as the middle class. In the tenements, New Yorkers sweetened their foods with just granulated sugar and molasses—none of the honey, maple syrup, and brown sugar used by the more affluent.

The austerity of New York's poor and unskilled can be glimpsed in the money-saving tips and daily menus collected by Caroline Goodyear, a social worker who spent three months interviewing charity-dependent women.[39] Among the things they taught her were how to stretch a food budget by purchasing cracked eggs, how to recycle leftover soup meat as hash or croquettes, and how to use sweetened condensed milk to spare the costs of sugar and butter.

The menus that Goodyear published represented the meals prepared over the course of one week by a thirty-seven-year-old woman who worked part time as an office cleaner. She cooked for a husband, four children, and an elderly lodger. On a mid-June Sunday in 1905, the woman fixed for her household a breakfast of pork chops accompanied by bread, butter, and tea. For the midday meal, she served corned beef, cabbages, and potatoes. Everyone revisited the beef served cold that evening. Breakfast the following Wednesday

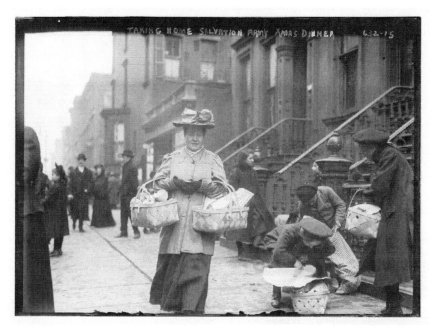

PHOTO 4.3
"Woman Carrying Baskets—Salvation Army Christmas Dinner, New York" (c. 1908).
While children eagerly inspect food baskets, a lady from the tenements totes hers home.
(Photograph by Bain News Service. Courtesy of the George Grantham Bain Collection
[LC-DIG-ggbain-03076], U.S. Library of Congress, Prints and Photographs Division.)

consisted of just bread and tea. There was ten cents worth of cheese for lunch, and in the evening the household had beans cooked with tomatoes. Favorite dishes included Italian vegetable pie (layers of potatoes, onions, and tomatoes with chopped meat), lyonnaise eggs (see recipe 4.3), and stewed tripe. Often what the family ate depended on what the oldest boy was able to acquire from wholesale grocers. Several grocers were in the habit of giving him the remains of canned and other packaged foods that were offered to customers as samples earlier that day. The boy's family recalled one particularly lucky day that climaxed with a feast after he came home with nine opened cans of salmon courtesy of a friendly wholesaler.

RECIPE 4.3

LYONNAISE EGGS

The family whose menus Caroline Goodyear chronicled may have been in unfortunate straits, but its members apparently preferred dishes possessing more character than simple plates of meat and potatoes. The lyonnaise eggs mentioned as a household favorite implied good taste. The name refers to the French city of Lyon, a place often acclaimed as the world capital of gastronomy.

For this recipe, we again turn to Maria Parloa (see recipe 4.2). Her instructions for making lyonnaise eggs appeared in *Miss Parloa's Kitchen Companion*.[1] Parloa spent time in France learning French cuisine firsthand, and her cookbooks contained many French recipes. While living for a time in New York City, she worked as a volunteer with women who made the crowded tenements their homes. She believed it was important to teach immigrants how to cook in their new and unfamiliar environment.[2] Here, in her own words, is the recipe for lyonnaise eggs that she may have taught:

If half a dozen eggs are to be cooked, use also two table-spoonfulls of butter, one of flour, one of chopped onion, three gills[3] of milk (one and one half pints), half a teaspoonful of salt, one-eighth of a teaspoonful of pepper, and half a cupful of grated bread crumbs. Cook the butter and onion slowly for ten minutes; then add the flour, and cook until the mixture becomes smooth and frothy, stirring all the while. Gradually add the milk, and cook for three minutes, stirring during the first minute. Add the salt and pepper. Pour the sauce into a deep plate that has been heated for the purpose. Carefully break the eggs into this plate, and cover them with the bread crumbs. Place in a moderately hot oven, and cook for four minutes. Serve the eggs in the dish in which they are cooked. If a strong flavor of onion be disagreeable, the sauce may be strained when it is poured upon the heated plate; the bits of onion being thus kept back.[4]

NOTES

1. Maria Parloa, *Miss Parloa's Kitchen Companion: A Guide for All Who Would Be Good Housekeepers* (Boston: Estes and Lauriat, 1887).

2. Anne-Marie Rachman, "Miss Parloa: Maria Parloa (September 25, 1843–August 21, 1909)," *Feeding America: The Historic American Cookbook Project*, Digital and Multimedia Center, Michigan State University Libraries, http://digital.lib.msu.edu/projects/cookbooks/html/authors/author_parloa.html.

3. One gill equals a half cup.

4. Parloa, *Miss Parloa's Kitchen Companion*, 409–10.

COMPARING NUTRITIONAL VALUES

Table 4.3 compares nutritional values derived from the dietaries described above. The upper half of the table concerns nutrition from animal products. The lower half of the table shows values specific to vegetable items in addition to values for total protein, fat, and energy. The last three columns in the lower half of the table indicate dietary variety over periods of seven, ten, and fourteen days.

Across the board, the table reveals higher values associated with middle-class standing. This is immediately evident by comparing the row labeled "Middle Class" with the row for "NYC Poor" under the seasonal heading "Winter." The values for spring bring skilled and semi-skilled Chicagoans into the picture. Here we see that the energy content of diets averaged higher among skilled workers than unskilled and averaged higher still among members of the middle class. Energy demands were likely the reverse. In other words, members of the middle class, on average, almost certainly spent less energy per day than skilled laborers, who in turn probably expended less energy per day than the unskilled.

Comparing the data for the households of skilled laborers to those of the unskilled suggests that the former used their limited resources to somewhat

Table 4.3. Average Nutritional Values by Season and Social Class

SEASON and SOCIAL CLASS	ANIMAL PRODUCTS (g/m/d)	ANIMAL PROTEIN (g/m/d)	% ENERGY ANIMAL FAT	% ENERGY ANIMAL	% BUDGET ANIMAL
FALL					
Middle Class		65	31	43	
NYC Poor	524	60	33	45	67
WINTER					
Middle Class	903	68	36	46	68
NYC Poor	430	44	27	37	59
SPRING					
Middle Class	849	65	31	43	58
Chicago Working Class		66	38	42	59
NYC Poor	534	55	26	39	57
SUMMER					
NYC Poor	738	63	32	46	58

SEASON and SOCIAL CLASS	VEGETABLE PRODUCTS (g/m/d)	TOTAL PROTEIN (g/m/d)	TOTAL FAT (g/m/d)	TOTAL ENERGY (Cal/m/d)	DIETARY VARIETY 7d	10d	14d
FALL							
Middle Class		109	134	3430			
NYC Poor	863	106	124	3175		27	
WINTER							
Middle Class	985	109	145	3393	30	33	31
NYC Poor	702	87	81	2461		24	
SPRING							
Middle Class	1002	107	123	3332		41	35
Chicago Working Class		119	138	3068	26		
NYC Poor	769	92	96	2733		28	
SUMMER							
NYC Poor	953	105	120	2987		28	

better advantage. The table shows that during the spring, all three classes allocated approximately the same percentage of their food dollars to items derived from animal sources. However, within their limited means, skilled workers were able to closely match or exceed middle-class intakes of animal protein, animal fat, total fat, and total protein. The families of the poor and unskilled came nowhere close to matching the intakes of members of the middle class, except during harvest season ("Fall" in the table), when food prices generally were at their lowest.

Table 4.3 indicates that, by and large, the middle class's nutritional advantage was due to the sheer quantity of food consumed. The table lists the average weights of both animal and vegetable items consumed per day. Considering the values for spring and adding animal and vegetable foodstuffs together reveals that while poor New Yorkers were consuming food at an average of 1,303 g/m/d (approximately 3 lb.), middle-class householders were putting it away at an average rate of 1,851 g/m/d (or about 1 lb. more food per day). Similarly, members of the middle class took in approximately one–and–three-quarters times the amount of meat and dairy products consumed by unskilled, working-class families. To its further advantage, the middle class as represented here benefited from greater dietary variety, eating nine to thirteen more foods over a period of ten days than people living in the tenements of New York.

Looking exclusively at winter's average intakes, the differences appear even greater. At this time of year, poor New Yorkers ate at an average rate of 1,132 g/m/d. Food consumption among representative middle-class households averaged 1,888 g/m/d. With regard to energy, the disparity was close to 1,000 Cal/m/d in favor of the middle class. Besides that, middle-class professionals took in an average of 12 g/m/d more protein. All of this supports the conventional understanding that during the Gilded Age, poverty imposed nutritional deprivations, but whether we can legitimately speak of a hunger problem remains open to question.

ANNUAL EBBS AND FLOWS

C. F. Langworthy, Atwater's successor at the OES, reflected on the many studies his office supported over the years. He saw in them no reason to regard hunger as a major problem in the United States.[40] Richard Hooker, writing many years later and from a broader historical perspective, held a less sanguine view.[41] As he interpreted the record, malnutrition posed an endemic problem. It troubled children in impoverished neighborhoods throughout the country. There were, in addition, economic depressions bringing recurrent episodes of hunger to American cities. Outside of urban areas, chronic deprivation pestered former slaves, white sharecroppers, and western farmers. Harvey Levenstein expressed a more cautious assessment.[42] He drew attention to the labor elite's ability to purchase the canned goods and bottled milk needed to bridge the naturally occurring scarcities of winter and spring. The poor had a hard time, but in his opinion they did not suffer frank hunger. City residents at worst had to subsist on a monotonous diet of potatoes, cabbage, turnips, perhaps some pickles, and a little milk. Folks in small towns and on farms could buy many of the same foods, including canned goods. Home canning also presented an option. Still, undependable transportation and a lack of ready cash created problems. These issues left many communities vulnerable to annual brushes with hunger.

The Rural South

Two types of annual hunger troubled the rural South. The first, which was specific to cotton-growing regions, occurred as regular episodes of protein-energy undernutrition. These episodes descended upon tenant farmers and plantation laborers in late autumn or early winter and ended with the arrival of spring. The Tuskegee families described in chapter 3 experienced this sort of seasonal hunger. A second type of hunger swept over areas of the South during the warm months of late spring and continued into the summer. It involved both a lack of niacin (vitamin B_3) in local diets and a deficiency of tryptophan, an amino acid that the body converts into niacin.[43] This problem eventually led to a great epidemic of pellagra, which persisted as a major public health menace well beyond the Atwater era. Charles Wait captured the nutritional pulse underlying this debilitating and potentially lethal disease during his Maryville, Tennessee, investigations (see chapter 2).

Cotton and the Postharvest Dead Season

Dorothy Dickins carried out a major study of food consumption among African American cotton farmers in Yazoo–Mississippi River delta just prior to the Great Depression.[44] Her assistants, black women native to the area, gathered information from eighty households during the months of Febru-

ary and March. This situated the project astride two major seasons of the
year on the agricultural calendar. Dickins's February inquiries documented
nutrition during the delta's so-called dead season. The records that her
assistants made in March depicted diet and nutrition to be an enormous
nutritional pulse. Its flow began on the very first of March. From that day
forward, until all of the cotton had been picked, families took three meals a
day. These meals consisted mostly of fresh fish, salt pork, flour, rice, cornmeal, dried peas, cane syrup, lard, and cabbage served in quantities sufficient to provide an average of 3,046 Cal/m/d. Nutrition began to ebb with
the conclusion of the crop in November. By February, it receded to its lowest
point, and most folks were down to just two meals a day. Many households
were reduced to eating no more than three foods—typically rice, beans, and
cornbread—over the course of a week.

Chances were that even those who made money on the previous year's crop
had to make do for some weeks on scant rations. Rarely were proceeds from
the previous year's crop sufficient to cover debts, and if money owed to landlords was not burden enough, there were shopkeepers in nearly every town
and village tempting people to buy sewing machines, fancy clocks, and other
expensive items on credit. These purchases were repossessed, often within a
matter of weeks.[45] In the meantime, a visitor might stumble upon the proud
owner of a new organ who was otherwise so bereft of household goods that
his family's tableware consisted of a single fork.[46]

The delta's great annual pulse from plenty to want and back again was
entirely artificial and completely at the service of cotton culture. Until it
came time to plant and tenants needed to muster sufficient energy to begin,
landlords neither advanced cash nor made credit available to purchase food.
Then, in an eye blink, on the precise day that the cotton season traditionally
got under way, supplies and provisions became available to everyone ready
to put in a crop.[47]

Researchers a generation earlier observed a similar regime at Tuskegee.[48]
There dietary records captured the nutritional upsurge mandated by spring
planting. The cotton farmers studied during the winter months subsisted
on an average of around 3,000 Cal/m/d. The average energy content of
food consumed by families once planting began in the spring swelled to
nearly 3,900 Cal/m/d. The dietaries show that about the time workers were
expected to plant, they were able to purchase more bacon than in previ-

ous months. Sugar and syrup consumption increased by nearly 75 percent. Cornmeal consumption rose only slightly, but the purchase of wheat flour jumped almost fourfold. The average protein intake ebbed and flowed in sync with energy. Total protein amounted to 65 g/m/d while spring planting was in progress, with 23 g/m/d coming from animal sources, largely eggs and milk. By December, chilly temperatures ended egg production and sharply curtailed milk supply. As a result, the animal-derived protein content of diets fell, on average, to a mere 7 g/m/d. Farmers began slaughtering their pigs about this time of year, raising the average intake to about 15 g/m/d. Nevertheless, overall protein consumption was exceedingly low by world standards. Indeed, the average intake of Italian beggars surpassed that of tenant farmers between growing seasons.[49]

The Pellagra Season

Maryville, Tennessee, was typical of areas in the South that were troubled annually by low protein intakes during the spring and summer months (see chapter 2). By comparison, autumn and winter were relatively bountiful. Ample supplies of cornmeal, wheat flour, and sweet potatoes during harvest season provided plenty of energy for a workforce made up primarily of manual laborers. Intakes for the fall averaged over 3,800 Cal/m/d, a prodigious quantity even by early twentieth-century American standards. Protein intake averaged 87 g/m/d. Just 21 g/m/d came from animal sources, but that was three times Tuskegee's fall average.

Eating habits changed once the temperature dropped below freezing. On the one hand, people increased their consumption of both beef and pork. On the other hand, they used somewhat less cornmeal, wheat flour, and other cereals. In addition, there were slightly fewer white potatoes on the table. Homemakers compensated by serving more sweet potatoes and turnips and by preparing a lot more cabbage, including sauerkraut. At the same time, the consumption of dairy products rose drastically. The use of fresh milk climbed from a fall average of approximately 15 g/m/d to about 145 g/m/d. This may have been due to cooler ambient temperatures during the fall, which made milk safer to drink than during the hot summer months (see below). Butter consumption declined in cold weather, but buttermilk use more than doubled. Altogether, dairy foods helped keep winter energy intakes relatively high—indeed, on average, just 3 percent less than during the fall.

Steep drops took place once spring arrived. Energy intake fell by more than 15 percent (see chapter 2). Total protein consumption declined by nearly the same number of percentage points. Protein from animal sources dropped by around 50 percent. Dairy consumption fell by an estimated 50 percent as well, with fresh milk almost completely disappearing from inventories. One Maryville household took in a scant 61 g/m/d of total protein. Later in the year, another household took in just 54 g/m/d, a mere 3 g/m/d above the World Health Organization's safe level of protein intake for an OES man-unit.[50] At nearby Crooked Creek, summer dietaries uncovered two households below a safe level of protein intake and three perilously close to it. Situations like these set the stage for pellagra.

Charles Wait, the chemist responsible for the Maryville dietaries, did not report seeing pellagra, even though the disease was soon to become common-place throughout the South. The initial cases in Tennessee were diagnosed in 1909, the very year Wait's research was published.[51] The next year more than one hundred cases were counted throughout the state. By 1911, the disease was widespread and creating alarm in many communities. Physicians quickly recognized it as a seasonal malady strongly associated with rural poverty.[52] Every year new cases began to show up in March. They peaked in June and by the end of October ceased to appear.

The disease made its presence known through a succession of symptoms, including the so-called 3 Ds—dermatitis, diarrhea, and dementia. Some cases culminated in death. Doctors discovered that pellagra could be cured by feeding victims a wholesome diet, but it was not until 1937 that the dis-ease was identified as a vitamin-deficiency condition. We now know that the disorder stems from diets poor in niacin (nicotinic acid), a B-complex vitamin present in foods and produced in the body from tryptophan, an amino acid found in most proteins.[53]

Pellagra investigator Joseph Goldberger and his associates suspected nu-tritional involvements as early as 1916. They studied food consumption in a number of cotton-mill villages in South Carolina.[54] Within a year, Goldberg-er's team discovered a key difference between villages with relatively high rates of pellagra and those having only a few cases. Compared to highly pellagrous villages, those relative immune to the disease consumed greater quantities of meat and dairy products. Researchers noted, too, that the appearance and disappearance of pellagra cases corresponded to the annual pulse of meat and dairy consumption. Mill workers, like folks throughout the South, ate most of their fresh meats during the cooler months. As the days grew warmer and meat storage became more challenging, supplies decreased and prices rose. Meat consumption in the warm climate of South Carolina began to drop off in some homes as early as February and in others as late as May. About the same time (March through April), the consumption of dairy products reached its yearly low. This coincidence, clearly visible in the Maryville data, had a negative effect on niacin availability by all but eliminating two important sources of tryptophan from the diets of the poor. The situation became acute after 1906, when commercial millers succeeded in removing the germ from corn. Their intent was to extend the shelf life of cornmeal. The unintended consequence was to reduce the tryptophan and its niacin equivalent in milled maize by about 50 percent.[55] This was the last straw for folks too poor to afford fresh meat or dairy products. Marginal insufficiencies became acute deficiencies, and annual epidemics of pellagra resulted.[56]

The Urban North

Working-class residents of northern cities faced their nutritional challenge during the cold-weather months. Dietaries conducted in Chicago revealed that just as temperatures were apt to turn bitterly cold, average energy intake declined by nearly 10 percent (from 3,400 to 3,141 Cal/m/d). Total protein intake at the same time slumped by almost 15 percent. Among poor American-born New Yorkers, winter brought the same drop in protein consumption and a decline of more than 20 percent in the energy content of diets.[57] This left households with just 2,461 Cal/m/d, a value difficult to imagine as adequate, particularly at a time when people lived in barely heated or unheated rooms and getting from place to place normally meant walking. But sufficient or not, intakes varied from house to house by little more than 350 Cal/m/d, and winter's mean value fell well within the range reported from Chicago (see chapter 5). This makes it reasonable to believe that a substantial number of poverty-stricken New Yorkers wintered on less than 2,500 Cal/m/d.

Explaining why winter energy intakes may have been so low among unskilled laborers brings up patterns of unemployment and underemployment. Slowdowns and layoffs in construction, transportation, and other industries sensitive to the cold and snow impinged on manual laborers more than anyone else. This rendered otherwise steady incomes fitful. A New York City trucker whose family's midwinter food consumption was studied for a period of ten days earned a mere two dollars during that time.[58] His wife, a janitor, did somewhat better, but a third member of the household, a cousin, worked only part time. Another household head who worked as a longshoreman made a little more than three dollars over the course of ten days. His son did a little better as a printer's assistant, but it was the longshoreman's wife who covered the rent thanks to her job as a housekeeper for an apartment building. The chief breadwinner for a third household that was studied for ten days failed to find any work whatsoever. His wife took in a little money doing laundry. His son help out on a truck wagon, but the family had to buy food by the meal and ate mostly stale bread.

To make matters worse for families like these, every year, just as the opportunities for earning income were diminishing, food prices went up. This was particularly true in New York City, where bringing down food costs during the winter was one of the main reasons put forward in favor of speeding up railroad construction.[59] As food prices rose in response to falling temperatures, total consumption among the households studied by OES fieldworkers dropped by nearly 300 g/m/d (approximately 10 oz.). The dietaries show that people in the tenements ate almost 20 percent less beef, 40 percent less pork, and 60 percent less fish by weight. The purchase of cooking fats and oils declined by an average of 40 percent. Households cut back on the use of refined sugars, on average, by one-third. Carrots, leeks, and parsnips, popular items on the fall table, were found less often (or not at all) during winter inventories.

However, a few foods appeared more often in the winter than in the autumn. There was more cabbage for dinner, and the use of cereals, dried beans, and potatoes rose to offset, at least partially, the energy losses brought about by the decreased consumption of fats and sugars. To answer to protein needs, egg consumption nearly doubled. Milk consumption also increased. Paradoxically, the average intake of animal carbohydrates declined, but this was probably due to less use of condensed milk, a product that contains nearly twice the carbohydrates found in fresh milk.

After a hard winter, spring brought about a reversal. The New York data indicate a rebound in energy intake of roughly 18 percent. Unskilled working-class households on Chicago's West Side experienced a 13 percent bounce. The protein content of working-class meals increased in both cities as well.

Families ate more meat. Indeed, beef purchases returned to autumn levels. Total fat intake rose by 25 percent in Chicago and 40 percent in New York City. Compared to winter, greater quantities of bacon, lard, salt pork, and suet entered people's diets; the same for olive oil and olive oil mixtures.

Once summer arrived, the average fuel values of diets turned around and again declined. The OES's data for New York City's tenement households show less meat consumption and less use of cooking fats. Diets included more vegetables and fruits. In addition, households consumed more dairy products, including fresh milk.

Milk in late nineteenth-century cities usually was bought from street vendors by the ladle. Summer brought abundant supplies and lower prices, but at the same time the danger of milk-borne illnesses increased. Not that milk was ever completely safe to drink. During the Gilded Age, urban dairymen often kept diseased cows that gave milk so peculiar vendors could not sell it without adulteration. However, what made milk especially dangerous during the summer was the increased risk of bacterial contamination because of higher ambient temperatures and lack of refrigeration. Bad milk resulted in "summer complaint" or "summer diarrhea," a disease that took the lives of countless children every year. People generally recognized the danger and chose canned condensed milk when they could afford it.

The poor were not the only Americans to experience seasonal fluctuations in nutrition during the Gilded Age. To a lesser extent, skilled and semi-skilled workers felt the same pulses as their less fortunate compatriots. Middle-class Americans also experienced annual ups and downs. These, however, ran counter to those faced by the working class.

The counterpoints can be appreciated by looking again at table 4.3. Notice that among the New York City poor, consumption of both animal and vegetable products dropped off sharply from fall to winter and rose again in the spring. The same was true for protein, fat, and total energy; intakes declined in winter and increased again afterward. For middle-class households, however, the pattern was different. Protein intake among the middle class remained fairly steady from season to season, while fat consumption rose dramatically during the winter. This probably accounts for the absence of any marked reduction in the average fuel value of diets transitioning from autumn into winter. Basically, it would appear that the middle class added fat to their winter fare by substantially increasing the proportion of their food budget devoted to meat and dairy products. For the working class, once winter arrived and vegetable prices rose significantly, meat and dairy spending, as a proportion of the food budget, contracted.

Ultimately, this creates the impression of a middle class effectively adjusting its nutrition to winter conditions by increasing its reliance on foods from animal sources and especially from items rich in fat and, consequently, high in fuel value. Among working-class families, winter brought more beans, cereals, and potatoes to the table, but not enough to offset declines in the consumption of animal fats and carbohydrates and, thereby, to maintain energy intakes at autumn levels. Worse yet, protein intake also dropped off going into winter, just as the annual incidence of various respiratory infections, including influenza, reached its height, and those who fell ill needed the protein to overcome their disease and repair damaged tissues. The problem essentially came down to seasonal price increases that most working-class families could not afford.

SEASONAL HUNGER AND ITS CONSEQUENCES

There exists physical evidence that during the Gilded Age, American workers in northern states were significantly undernourished for at least part of the year. The evidence is anthropometric—which is to say, the evidence resides in comparative measurements of the human body.

Scientists investigating aspects of human growth and development have been keenly interested in anthropometric data for generations. More recently, an anthropometric history has emerged from the efforts of economic historians who found in modern growth and development studies a way to compare living standards and determine how they changed following industrialization.[60]

The groundbreaking idea was to use measurements of adult stature over time as a means to infer relative well-being. Inferences about well-being based on average adult height rest on substantial evidence that undernutrition and disease negatively affect human growth. Genetics establish growth potentials; the cumulative effects of diet and health-related experiences, particularly during childhood, determine to what extent those potentials are realized. Growth rates are exceedingly sensitive to nutritional deprivation. Insufficient protein stunts growth. Too little energy from carbohydrates and fat produces the same effect by causing protein to be diverted from tissue building and used instead as fuel. A bout with disease can also retard growth by redirecting protein to tissue repair. Full height may still be achieved if subsequent nutrition is good.

But prolonged or repeated episodes of deprivation, such as seasonal hunger, eventually result in a reduction of average height among adults owing to unfulfilled growth potential.[61]

Examining nineteenth-century records of male stature, anthropometric historians learned that working-class men, on average, attained significantly shorter statures than men in the upper ranks of society. Such deficits were greater during the nineteenth and early twentieth centuries than in subsequent years. Thus, military records showing average heights by occupation varied only slightly among World War II recruits.[62] Earlier on, between the years 1870 and 1930, national guardsmen who earned their livings as professionals stood almost an inch taller than their comrades-in-arms who were employed as wage laborers.[63]

To the extent that such disparities can be attributed directly to undernutrition, the lion's share of damage most likely was inflicted during the winter, when the gap in average energy intake between the middle class and the unskilled laborers approached 1,000 Cal/m/d (see table 4.3). A wintertime disadvantage in an average protein intake of around 15 g/m/d, not to mention substantial class differences continuing into spring, must have impeded the growth of working-class children even more. This should lay to rest Levenstein's contention that winter for working-class families in cities was little more than a period of dietary monotony.[64] OES data for New York City, no less than that recorded for the Black Belt and the mountains of eastern Tennessee, all describe a nutritional roller coaster destined annually to descend into a deep trough during a certain season of the year—in effect, a genuine hunger season, one as real and as pernicious as many of those documented for parts of Africa throughout the latter half of the twentieth century.[65]

Immigrants' Diets

Donna Gabaccia views the period from the late nineteenth through the early twentieth centuries as a uniquely conservative time in American culinary history.[1] During the colonial era, people had been open to experimentation and change, but by the turn of the twentieth century most Americans were either unwilling or unable to try new foods. The unwilling identified strongly with their communities and cherished their accustomed food habits. The unable were prevented by their poverty from changing the way they ate. Together custom and privation collaborated to define seven major variations on the meat-rich, white-floured, heavily sweetened standard American diet. Gabaccia identifies the variants as northern European, southern European, Asian, Mexican American, and native southern (or African American).[2] Previous chapters dealt with examples of mainstream American, the American South, and Mexican American diets. This chapter addresses food consumption among immigrants from Europe. Their dietaries attest to stark differences in nutrition among various nationalities. In addition, the dietaries indicate changes in diet as fortunes improved and lives became increasingly Americanized. This gives one pause and reason to think carefully about characterizing this period as conservative.

EUROPEAN IMMIGRANTS

Dietaries undertaken in Gilded Age America documented the eating habits of immigrants representing thirteen distinct European nationalities.[3] Of

these, German American groups received the most attention.[4] This chapter
examines eating and drinking among these and several other sets of European
immigrants, including those from Bohemia, Great Britain, Ireland, Italy, and
Russia's Jewish communities.[5]

The eating habits of European Americans generally had much in common.
Indeed, the typical diets of most of them shared a constellation of twenty-two
core foodstuffs. Six of these, listed in table 5.1 as "Primary Core in All," were
universal among all of the ethnicities covered in this chapter. Eight counted as
primary core foods among *most* European Americans. Another eight qualified as at least secondary core foods among *most*. The bottom row of the table,
labeled "Included in Most," represents those items that would qualify as peripheral to a typical European American diet. The items listed showed up in
just two of the seven typical diets considered here. The specific, individual
character of each of the diets took shape mainly through the addition and
subtraction of primary and secondary core foods.

Italian Americans

Italian immigration to the United States began in earnest in the 1860s.
It peaked in 1900, but Italians continued to arrive in substantial numbers
until the outbreak of World War I. The overwhelming majority of Italian
immigrants came from places in southern Italy, especially from towns and
villages situated in Abruzzo, Calabria, Campania, and Sicily. Many of these
immigrants were recruited as manual laborers. Large numbers signed on to
work in mines and mills. Countless thousands of these recruits and their de-
pendents found themselves packed together in dilapidated areas of big cities,
previously occupied by other nationalities but more recently converted into
"little Italies."[6]

The earliest records of Italian American food consumption were created
in 1892 under the auspices of Philadelphia's College Settlement Association.[7]
Robert Coit Chapin provided the era's final look when, in 1906, he published
a pair of household food budgets carried out in New York City.[8] Prior to
that, the investigators had managed to complete just one study of an Italian
household in New York, in effect echoing the near-total failure that occurred
in Chicago a few years earlier.[9]

Table 5.1. Foods Commonly Part of European American Diets about 1900

	Meat and Dairy	Grains and Dried Legumes	Fats, Oils, Sugars, and Starches	Roots and Tubers	Other Vegetables	Fruits and Misc.
Primary Core in All	fresh beef[1] egg milk		sugar	potato onion[2]		
Primary Core in Most	veal[3] fresh pork[4] fresh fish[5]	wheat flour wheat bread	butter lard		cabbage	
Core in Most	ham[6] cheese[7]	oats[8] rye bread cake[9] beans			tomato[10]	apple[11]
Included in Most	beef liver bologna pork sausage bacon chicken mutton[12] sardine	rice barley roll cracker pie[13] beer	suet[14] cocoa	carrot turnip	cucumber	banana orange lemon prune fruit jelly[15]

1. various cuts
2. fresh and dried
3. diverse cuts
4. various cuts
5. assorted species
6. variety of types
7. assorted types
8. includes rolled oat and meal
9. different kinds
10. fresh and canned
11. fresh and dried
12. various cuts
13. variety of fillings
14. includes ordinary beef fat
15. various kinds

The plan in Chicago had been to inventory a substantial number of households. Settlement workers fanned out around Hull House, less than a mile southwest of Union Station, where they approached dozens of families of Italian immigrants and asked them to participate in a study. Many of them agreed at first, but almost as soon as the counting and weighing began, nearly everyone who had signed up for the project dropped out.[10] Some called it quits the very first time a fieldworker showed up and began asking questions. Most families tolerated the intrusions for a day or two. Only four families

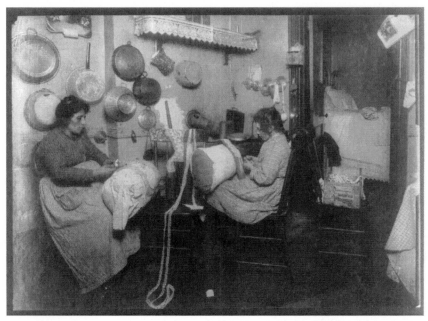

PHOTO 5.1

"Mrs. Palontona and 13-Year-Old Daughter, Michaeline, Working on 'Pillow-Lace' in Dirty Kitchen of Their Tenement Home . . ." (1911). Tenement kitchens often doubled as income-earning workrooms. (Photograph by Lewis Wickes Hine. Courtesy of the records of the National Child Labor Committee [LC-USZ62-29124], U.S. Library of Congress, Prints and Photographs Division.)

put up with the daily data gathering for a full week. Three of these families included men out of work. The fourth consisted of three brothers, one of them a sixteen-year-old who kept house for the other two.

Because most of the people asked to participate in the Chicago study quickly dropped out, the few who cooperated throughout the entire project cannot be called entirely "typical." Nevertheless, one thing that proved characteristic from one household to the next was a remarkable lack of concern about the cost of food. Ellen Richards and Amelia Shapleigh's data from Philadelphia show that food costs for Italian Americans ran well above those of other ethnic groups.[11] Chapin's standards-of-living survey involving 318 New York City households uncovered a similar pattern, with Italian Americans in three out of five income groups spending a greater portion of their household budget on food than any of seven other nationalities.[12] Outlays for vegetables and fruits ran especially high across all income brackets.[13] Wine, beer, and other alcoholic beverages showed up as other relatively expensive tastes.[14]

W. O. Atwater and A. P. Bryant blamed the high cost of the typical Italian American diet on an obstinate attachment to the traditional culture of the Old Country.[15] Commodities such as olive oil had been cheap in Italy. The same products were often dear in the United States. This did not deter immigrants longing for familiar flavors. They insisted on buying their native oils, familiar cheeses, and other steeply priced imports. Families ate locally grown produce, but nevertheless the Italian American market basket often included such relatively expensive items as dandelion greens, parsley, and spinach instead of the less costly vegetables that Atwater and Bryant termed *indigenous*.[16]

Italians believed that the higher prices they paid were justified by the superior quality of their diet. In their opinion, they ate better than members of other nationalities, and generally speaking newcomers from Italy expressed little interest in trying other peoples' foods.[17] This created the impression that Italians disliked foreign dishes. Word circulated that they dreaded going to the hospital for medical help and that they avoided seeking employment outside of their own neighborhoods because of the unfamiliar foods they might have to eat.[18] Regardless of whether this was true, it seems fair to say that no nationality other than the Chinese clung with greater tenacity to their native cuisine.[19]

A typical Italian American diet based on food inventories conducted during the winter and spring differed from the standard European American model in several ways. To start with, and not surprisingly, Italians made macaroni a primary core food.[20] Sausage, olive oil, and spinach were unique secondary items.[21] The hams and apples generally popular among other European immigrants were not often seen in Italian American kitchens of this period.

Core meat and dairy products were not consumed in particularly large quantities. Most families from southern Italy were practically vegetarians prior to emigrating because they could ill afford meat. Some were unable to buy spaghetti. Before coming to America, a typical meal might consist of a piece of bread dipped in olive oil and salt, or perhaps a bean and cabbage soup dressed with a bit of lard or a few drops of olive oil.[22] Poorly paid wage earners in Naples generally ate at small shops, where they could purchase a number of different kinds of macaroni and other "flour pastes."[23] Macaroni was a fairly common food on American tables by the mid-1890s, but at the time few Americans had heard of pizza, another Neapolitan dish. Atwater described it as dough "pressed in flat cakes baked with fat or cheese and tomatoes or with small fresh fish."[24]

Flour pastes and doughs, boiled and baked, and a variety of legumes, including dried beans, lentils, and peas, continued as the pillars of subsistence
among Italians in the United States. Pastas and legumes often wound up together in soups such as minestrone or pasta fagioli. Considered as individual
species, no particular legume ranked as a primary core food in the typical
Italian American diet, but taken together legumes were as central as white
bread and macaroni.

A number of foods of peripheral importance to the diet of Italian immigrants were not typically seen in other European American homes. Such products included beef tripe, oysters, salt fish, cornmeal, string beans, and various
nuts and olives. Cornmeal was exclusively Italian as far as immigrants were
concerned. It became polenta in the hands of Italian cooks, but it attracted no
interest from other new arrivals.

Table 5.2 displays average nutritional intakes for all of the sets of immigrants considered in this chapter and two non-European sets (French Canadian and Chinese) to be considered in the next chapter. For Italian American
households, the table serves to underscore how little emphasis meat and dairy
consumption received. Among those represented here, no other nationality
depended less on animal foods as sources of energy. What the table does not
show is the relatively small proportion of the food budget that was spent on
meat and dairy products. While other nationalities expended 60 percent more
of their food monies on such items, Italian households spent an average of just
50 percent, about the same percentage as Chinese immigrants.

Yet, in spite of having a diet in excess of 60 percent vegetable by weight,
Italian Americans consumed considerable quantities of fat. Households sampled by the OES generally drew approximately 35 percent of their total energy
from fat. Intakes averaged about 32 percent specifically from animal fat, much
of it consumed in the form of lard and cheese (see table 5.2). Most Italians
arrived in America with strong predilections toward both commodities. In
places like Abruzzo or Sicily, their appetites for animal fats generally out-
stripped their means.[25] The generally low cost of such fats in the United States
changed that and, as a result, radically altered the typical diet. Representative
data collected from mechanics in Naples, for example, show fat contributing
just 15 percent to a total energy supply that averaged just under 2,300 Cal/
m/d.[26] These values, compared to those for Italians living in the United States,
suggest that by emigrating from their native country, families increased the

ZUPPA DI FAGIUOLI

This recipe for bean soup came from Maria Gentile's *The Italian Cookbook*.[1] She wrote it to represent the home cooking that new immigrants brought with them to America.[2] This particular soup, according to Gentile, fell into a class of soups referred to as *Minestra di Magro* or "lean soup." This made it a Friday soup or a soup appropriate for any other day on which the Roman Catholic Church proscribed meat eating.

To make zuppa di fagiuoli, Maria started with a cup of dried beans—kidney, navy, or lima—and soaked them overnight. The next day she placed the beans, along with a pinch of baking soda, in a pot of cold water and brought it to a boil. She poured the water off and replaced it with fresh water. The pot was then returned to a boil and allowed to continue until the beans became tender.

In the meantime, Maria chopped a quarter of an onion, a clove of garlic, a sprig of parsley, and a stick of celery. These were combined in a pan and fried in a quarter cup of oil. Maria added salt and pepper at this point. When the chopped vegetables became slightly browned, she added two cups of water from the beans and a cup of tomatoes (fresh or canned). She brought all of this to a boil and added it to the cooked beans. If the beans were too liquid, they needed to be partially drained before adding the other ingredients. Maria sometimes served the soup as is. Other times she ran it through a sieve before serving. Croutons or triangles of dry toast, she thought, made an excellent addition.

NOTES

1. Maria Gentile, *The Italian Cook Book: The Art of Eating Well, Practical Recipes of the Italian Cuisine, Pastries, Sweets, Frozen Delicacies, and Syrups* (New York: Italian Cook Book Co., 1919), 9–10.

2. Anne-Marie Rachman, "*The Italian Cookbook*," *Feeding America: The Historic American Cookbook Project*, Digital and Multimedia Center, Michigan State University Libraries, http://digital.lib.msu.edu/projects/cookbooks/html/books/book_71.cfm.

Table 5.2. Average Nutritional Values for Diets of Nine Immigrant Groups

ETHNIC IDENTITY	Animal CHO (g/m/d)	Animal Protein (g/m/d)	% Energy Animal Fat	% Energy Animal Products
Italian	11	57	32	39
Russian Orthodox Jews	12	71	24	36
Russian Liberal Jews	19	96	26	41
Bohemian	22	87	30	44
Irish	14	74	33	44
British	15	78	32	43
German	19	63	30	42
French Canadians[1]	11	77	37	48
Chinese[2]	7	63	31	42
ETHNIC IDENTITY	Vegetable CHO (g/m/d)	Total Protein (g/m/d)	Total Fat (g/m/d)	Total Energy (Cal/m/d)
Italian	348	112	125	3120
Russian Orthodox Jews	399	121	87	2988
Russian Liberal Jews	411	153	106	3373
Bohemian	403	138	127	3553
Irish	400	117	137	3404
British	452	133	147	3767
German	362	112	114	3047
French Canadians[1]	369	121	166	3567
Chinese[2]	293	117	113	2760

1. Chicago residents only (see chapter 6)
2. San Francisco boarding house, light work (see chapter 6)

energy content of their diets by more than 35 percent (see table 5.2). At same time, they may have more than doubled their consumption of fat as measured by its contribution to energy intake.

Russian American Jews

Russian immigration to United States amounted to little more than a trickle prior to 1881. However, in that year it topped ten thousand new arrivals. By the end of the nineteenth century, Russian immigration to the United States would be averaging well over fifty thousand arrivals a year. Those emigrating were prompted by political repression, economic hardship, and religious persecution.[27] The majority of those persecuted were Jews. Escaping the 1881–1882 pogroms and various forms of harassment, Russian Jews fled to New York and other American cities.[28] Chicago became home to the largest population of Russian Jews in the Midwest, and almost immediately they reconstituted *shtetl* culture on the city's Near West Side.[29] A major center of community life emerged in the congested neighborhood around Maxwell Street, where the immigrants created a lively outdoor market.[30] It was in this neighborhood that OES scientists, who wondered about the nutritional consequences of the Jewish food habits, located their field studies.[31]

Orthodox Diets

Working with Bryant during the spring and fall of 1895, Atwater oversaw the collection of dietaries from ten Orthodox Jewish families, all settled in Chicago within the previous five years.[32] Family members ate and drank in full accordance with Judaism's dietary laws, which designated the consumption of pork and certain other meats as taboo. The laws also required ritual procedures when slaughtering animals, salting meat to remove blood, and cooking and serving meat and milk separately.

The Jews recruited for this study were very poor. By the time they arrived on Chicago's West Side, they could afford to rent nothing better than filthy basements and dark, windowless rooms. There they subsisted on a diet second only to the Italian's in its bias toward vegetables and fruits. Again, the practical necessity of subsisting mostly on vegetable products was something they had plenty of experience with before emigrating. A breakfast in Russia might have consisted of barley soup with oats; for dinner, perhaps some potatoes and milk or maybe some barley with peas or lima beans flavored with a speck of chicken fat. A morsel of pickled herring was viewed as a special treat.[33] The diet of even the most impoverished Jews in Gilded Age Chicago included more animal products than they could ever have imagined back home. Still, meals in Orthodox households contained considerably less animal content than other immigrants typically enjoyed.

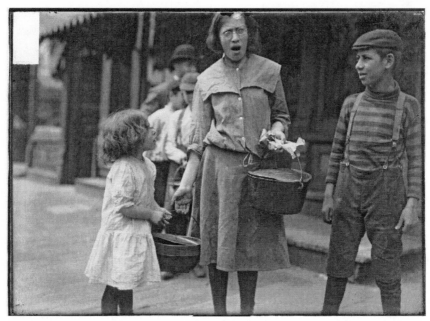

PHOTO 5.2
"Two Jewish Girls Carrying Pots of Food for the Sabbath" (1903). A newspaper photographer captured this street scene near Chicago's Maxwell Street Market. (Photograph by Chicago Daily News, Inc. Courtesy of the Chicago Daily News Negatives
Collection [DN-0001469], Chicago History Museum.)

Such was especially true of animal fat. Chicago's Orthodox averaged 36
percent of their energy intake from animal sources (see table 5.2), but for
the most part these were exceedingly lean. Beef fat was used sparingly. The
same was true of chicken fat. Homemakers purchased live chickens and
killed and dressed them according to Jewish custom, but they found little
fat on the carcasses. One family, for example, purchased fifteen pounds and
five ounces (seven kilograms) of chicken over the course of thirty-three
days. From that they garnered only about one gram of fat. The bottom line
was a diet in which animal fat contributed an average of just 24 percent of
a person's energy supply (see table 5.2). Fats in total amounted to not much
more. Energy intake was relatively low among Orthodox Jews—an average
of less than 3,000 Cal/m/d (see table 5.2). This stood considerably below
average for immigrants generally.[34]

RECIPE 5.2

BORSHT AND OTHER BEET SOUPS

The recipes presented here are Florence Greenbaum's.[1] They relate just a few of the many traditional ways in which Russian and other Eastern European Jews prepared beets for their families' enjoyment. Greenbaum studied chemistry and diet at Hunter College in New York City.[2] She went on to teach cooking and domestic science at the Young Women's Hebrew Association. By the time she published *The International Jewish Cook Book* in 1918, she was lecturing at other institutions in the city under the auspices of the Bureau of Jewish Education.

The full title of Greenbaum's work, *The International Jewish Cook Book: 1600 Recipes according to the Jewish Dietary Laws with the Rules for Kashering: The Favorite Recipes of America, Austria, Germany, Russia, France, Poland, Roumania, Etc., Etc.,* reflects both its orthodoxy and its enormous scope. Many of the recipes were treasured by Greenbaum's own family and had been handed down for several generations.[3]

Borsht: Florence Greenbaum's instructions for preparing borsht required but four sentences:

Take some red beetroots, wash thoroughly and peel, and then boil in a moderate quantity of water from two to three hours over a slow fire, by which time a strong red liquor should have been obtained. Strain off the liquor, adding lemon juice, sugar, and salt to taste, and when it has cooled a little, stir in sufficient yolks of eggs to slightly thicken it. May be used either cold or hot. In the latter case a little home-made beef stock may be added to the beet soup.[4]

Beet Soup—Russian Style: This recipe brings some sour cream to the beet liquor. Begin by cutting two small beets into strips, covering them with water, and cooking them until tender. Add citric acid (called "sour salt" at the grocery store) and a little

(*continued*)

RECIPE 5.2 (*continued*)

sugar to make the liquid sweet and sour. Add a little salt and three-quarters of a cup of sour cream. The dish should be served cold. Sweet cream may be used instead of sour cream. If doing so, add the cream, and while the liquid is still hot, pour it over the well-beaten yolks of two eggs. Keep the soup on the stove and stir constantly until the soup is thick and smooth. Then remove it from the stove and serve cold.[5]

Beet Soup—Russian Style (*Fleischig*): This recipe adds meat. It starts with one large beet, a half of pound of onions, and a one-pound piece of brisket of beef with fat. The beet and the onions both are cut into thick pieces and placed in a kettle with the fatty brisket. Everything is covered with water and set to cook slowly for about two hours. At that point, three-quarters of a cup of sugar and a little citric acid (sour salt) get added, making the liquid sweet and sour. Cook for another hour; season as desired and serve hot.[6]

NOTES

1. Florence Kreisler Greenbaum, *The International Jewish Cook Book: 1600 Recipes according to the Jewish Dietary Laws with the Rules for Kashering: The Favorite Recipes of America, Austria, Germany, Russia, France, Poland, Roumania, Etc., Etc.* (New York: Bloch, 1919).

2. Anne-Marie Rachman, "Florence Kreisler Greenbaum," *Feeding America: The Historic American Cookbook Project*, Digital and Multimedia Center, Michigan State University Libraries, http://digital.lib.msu.edu/projects/cookbooks/html/authors/author_greenbaum.html.

3. Ibid.

4. Greenbaum, *International Jewish Cook Book*, 14.

5. Ibid., 27.

6. Ibid., 14.

The diet of Orthodox Jews distinguished itself substantially from that of most European Americans (see table 5.1). On the animal side, there was the previously mentioned prohibition against pork. Distinctive additions to the primary core included "wienerwurst," chicken, smoked herring, cottage cheese, and sour cream. The wieners consisted of all-beef Vienna sausages, which became known as "hot dogs" some years later when they were served on buns. The cottage cheese went into cheese cakes, blintzes, and scores of other dishes. The sour cream was used in baking. It often accompanied potato pancakes and also was used to dress herring and other kinds of fish. On the grain and vegetable side, rye bread and apples qualified as primary foods; the same went for rice, lemons, and raisins. Unique additions to the secondary core consisted of beef suet, radishes, oranges, prunes, and various fruit jellies. Characteristic peripherals included ginger bread, beets, horseradish, pickles, vinegar, and soda water.

Liberal Diets

Atwater and Bryant referred to persons who identified themselves as Jewish but who did not adhere strictly to Judaic dietary rules as "unorthodox" or "liberal Jews."[35] Six household dietary studies conducted in Chicago and two cost-of-living studies—one carried out in New York City, the other in Boston—documented the eating habits of the unorthodox.[36]

Situations among these households varied considerably. Half of those in Chicago had left Russia within the previous five years. One was in considerable economic distress with six "puny, sickly, and irritable" children and a daily income of less than one dollar.[37] The head of another household found himself frequently unemployed. Male occupations included carpenter, street peddler, bicycle maker, school teacher, and musician. Among the women, one person folded shirts, another packed candies. A single mother supporting two children made neckties and earned extra income by preparing meals for a boarder.

The typical diet in these cases was not entirely unlike that of the Orthodox. Fish was positioned alongside beef as a primary food. Carp was important, but herring (fresh and smoked) and salmon (fresh and canned) were especially popular. Beef purchases excluded identifiable cuts from hindquarters, though homemakers showed no apparent concern about the origins of chopped beef.[38] Items not central to most European American diets but consumed in most non-Orthodox households were dried peas, apples, oranges, and prunes. Foods of secondary importance consisted of chicken, cottage cheese, and barley. Lemons and raisins, core foods in the typical Orthodox diet, were peripheral among nonconforming Jews. Dried beef, beef sausage, pork sausage, dairy cream, condensed milk, sour cream, aged cheese, and cream cheese were also of peripheral importance. Vegetable products in the peripheral category included prepared cereals, unleavened bread, prepared noodles, olive oil, beets, radishes, pickles, rhubarb, sauerkraut, wine, prepared soups, and soda water.

Nutritionally, the diets of non-Orthodox Jews contained more energy and more fat than the typical Orthodox diet (see table 5.2). Still, their energy content barely measured up to native Russian standards. The diet of a Moscow-area peasant had nearly the same fuel value, while the average energy intake among Moscow factory workers exceeded the Chicago average.[39] Total fat consumption, on the other hand, was relatively high (see table 5.2). Chicago's Russian Jewish Americans took in around a quarter of their food energy from animal fat. While this was far less than the average for most other European immigrant diets, it was two to three times greater than what Russians normally consumed in the Moscow area.[40]

Protein consumption also exceeded Moscow's averages by a long shot. For that matter, none of the other nationalities studied by Gilded Age nutritionists topped the average protein consumption recorded for Chicago's non-Orthodox Jews. This was achieved by dedicating a relatively large percentage of the typical food budget (68 percent) to the purchase of products from animal sources; the same was true for New York City, where Jews demonstrated considerable appetites for meat and fish.[41]

Bohemian Americans

Emigration from Bohemia, the modern Czech Republic for the most part, was especially heavy from about 1870 through 1890. Those who left were predominately small landowners and farmers, people who generally owned a house, a few pigs, and some other small stock. Their crops, raised mainly for subsistence, consisted of wheat and rye, various roots and tubers (potatoes, beets, onions, and turnips), and cabbage, the one leafy green that kept through the winter.[42] From these staples, Bohemians created a famously heavy cuisine constructed of meat dishes, potatoes, various breadkinds (dumplings and noodles included), and cabbage recipes. Country folk took nourishment from this fare four or five times a day.

Bohemians newly arrived in the United States remained true to their Old World food habits. In Chicago, this required spending an average of nearly 70 percent of a household's food budget on foods from animal sources. Bohemian budgets resembled the Russian Jews in this respect. But unlike the Jews, whose diets were relatively lean, Bohemian Americans favored fat. Animal fat plus large helpings of animal carbohydrates, stemming from a hearty appetite for milk and cheese, resulted in a diet in which meat and dairy items contributed, on average, 44 percent of the energy supply (see table 5.2). These estimates derive from twenty-six Chicago dietaries conducted during the winter of 1895 and spring of 1896 among families in a variety of economic circumstances.[43] Household income sources ranged from unskilled labor through various skilled and white-collar occupations.

Families patronized food markets catering specifically to Bohemian tastes. In these markets, shoppers were able to purchase ducks, rabbits, bologna, frankfurters, poppy seeds, and a number of other prized foods. Pork sausages, hams, and other cured pork products were in especially high demand. However, as for fresh meat, beef topped pork in most homes. Veal, too, was popular, but its status as a primary core food was limited to late winter and early spring, when it tended to be plentiful and cheap. The use of beef organ meats and bones, secondary core foods among Bohemians, was perpetual. Customers at Bohemian markets received gratis a quarter pound of beef liver and a six-ounce soup bone with the purchase of beef, no matter the quantity. Another meat-market tradition had the butcher flanked by a platter of chopped beef to one side and a platter of chopped pork to the other, mixing together the amounts that individual customers preferred. It was the same for milk and cream. Milk among Bohemian Americans meant skimmed milk. Milkmen sold cream separately, blending it with milk as requested. The proportion of cream depended on how much a customer wanted to pay.[44]

Breads and other things made from wheat flour, rye flour, and barley lent bulk to Bohemian cookery. Fieldworkers noted wheat flour in twenty-three kitchens, rye flour in nineteen. Wheat bread from the bakery was found in eleven households, rye bread in seven. Barley in granular form was used in ten households. Barley in the form of liquid bread—in other words, beer—was reported for fourteen households.[45]

The fruit and vegetable components of the Bohemian immigrants' typical diet were much the same as they were in the Old World. Chicago's Bohemians ate potatoes, onions, and cabbage during the late winter and spring and little else. Beets, carrots, and parsnips amounted to no more than peripheral items in the diet, but sauerkraut, apples, prunes, and lemons counted as secondary components. The fresh taste of lettuce came as a welcome change, and as winter gave way to spring, it, too, became a secondary core food.

Atwater and Bryant attached to their Bohemian dietaries information about immigrants' length of residence in the United States.[46] By comparing the eating habits of households new to the country with the eating habits of long-time residents, they hoped to develop an understanding of how diet and nutrition changed as a consequence of Americanization. Table 5.3 pursues this by distinguishing among immigrant Bohemian households located in the United States for less than ten years, immigrant Bohemian households located in the United States for more than ten years, and second-generation households headed by Bohemian couples who were born in the United States.[47]

Across the board, the table displays values that increase with length of residence in the United States. Beginning with first-generation immigrants with

Table 5.3.   Average Nutritional Values of Bohemian Diets by Length of Residence in the United States

YEARS LIVING IN USA	Animal CHO (g/m/d)	Animal Protein (g/m/d)	% Energy Animal Fat	% Energy Animal Products
< 10 Years	22	78	29	42
> 10 Years	23	96	32	47
Since Birth	23	115	37	52
YEARS LIVING IN USA	Vegetable CHO (g/m/d)	Total Protein (g/m/d)	Total Fat (g/m/d)	Total Energy (Cal/m/d)
< 10 Years	388	128	119	3469
> 10 Years	416	150	139	3706
Since Birth	413	175	181	4160

RECIPE 5.3

FRIED PORK TENDERLOIN

Marie Rosický (1854–1912) was born in Klatovy, Bohemia. She came to the United States at the age of thirteen. All of the women in her family had reputations as good cooks, which made her daughter Rose suspect that Marie inherited her culinary skills naturally.[1]

Marie wrote and originally published her *Bohemian-American Cookbook: Tested and Practical Recipes for American and Bohemian Dishes* in the Bohemian language. After Marie died, Rose Rosický decided to translate her mother's recipes into English, primarily as a service to the descendants of Bohemian immigrants who never learned to read Bohemian. Another prompt came from American housewives curious about Bohemian dishes but at a loss for finding authentic recipes.[2]

The recipe given here is exceedingly simple—so simple that some may regard it as an American dish. To Marie Rosický, American and simple went together in the kitchen. Most Americans, in her opinion, prepared only dishes that require little time and almost no labor.

The fried pork tenderloin from Rosický's cookbook offers a case in point. It proved so quick and easy that it essentially bypassed the American home kitchen to become the centerpiece of the tenderloin sandwich, a fast-food restaurant favorite unique to the Midwest. Mechanization, freezing, and deep-fat frying reduced preparation time to just a few minutes. Enclosing the fried tenderloin in a hamburger bun along with lettuce, tomato, and sauces covers much of the tenderloin's delicate taste. Nonetheless, Rosický's recipe attests to the truth of her belief that simple dishes properly prepared are as good as any.

To make fried pork tenderloin, begin by washing and trimming the tenderloin. After that, cut it into four pieces by slicing first lengthwise, then across. Pound each piece until it is completely

(*continued*)

RECIPE 5.3 (*continued*)

flattened. Dust the meat with salt, pepper, and flour. Dip each piece into a bowl of beaten eggs and then immediately into a bowl of bread crumbs to which a pinch of sage has been added. Fry the breaded meat in hot fat and serve immediately.

The pieces can be presented as pork schnitzels, accompanied, perhaps, by potatoes or *spätzle*, or they can be used to create your own rendition of the tenderloin sandwich.

NOTES

1. Marie Rosický, *Bohemian-American Cookbook: Tested and Practical Recipes for American and Bohemian Dishes (an English Language Translation of the Cook Book Published in the Bohemian Language and Compiled by Marie Rosický)*, 5th ed. (Omaha, NE: Automatic Printing Company, 1949), first published 1915.

2. Ibid.

---

less than a decade of American experience and culminating with American-born families, households consumed greater quantities of food containing increasing measures of energy, fat, and protein. Controlling for season corroborates the pattern. Looking at the spring months exclusively, American-born Bohemian households consumed, on average, 40 percent more food by weight than households that originated overseas. With respect to vegetable products alone, the dietaries indicate that Bohemian Americans ate roughly 70 percent more food by weight than their foreign-born counterparts. Potato consumption accounted for most of the difference. Also worth noting is the fact that American-born households used an average of about 30 percent more animal fat than immigrant households and consumed over 40 percent more vegetable fat. On average, Chicago's American-born Bohemians drew close to 40 percent of their total food energy from fat, much of it added to foods by frying them.

Irish Americans

Irish immigration to America began in the seventeenth century. At first, much of it involved Protestants from Ulster—the so-called Scots-Irish—many of whom headed directly for the Appalachians. By the 1820s, this had changed. From then on, most people arriving from Ireland were Catholics from the South and West, troubled by poverty and lured to America by reports of plenty of good-paying jobs. The Great Famine of the 1840s intensified immigration. Well over four and a half million Irish citizens made their way to the United States before the nineteenth century ended. Once they had landed, most of them settled in the great cities of the East and Midwest, unwilling or unable to move to less crowded areas.[48]

A total of nineteen dietary studies conducted in Chicago, New York, Philadelphia, and Pittsburgh tell of the eating habits of the Irish immigrants who arrived in the midst of America's Gilded Age.[49] These inquiries, all of them carried out in the 1890s, measured the diets of households in diverse circumstances. Individual situations ranged from jobless and frankly needy to fully employed and financially comfortable.

The typical diet of nearly one and all, irrespective of how well they were doing, included corned beef—otherwise referred to as "salt beef." This is a good food with which to begin a discussion of Irish American eating habits because of an apparent disconnect. On the one hand, there are repeated observations by early nutritionists of corned beef in family kitchens, and on the other hand, there is the position taken by culinary historian Hasia Diner in her highly regarded book *Hungering for America*.[50] The book contains two chapters about Irish and Irish American foodways; yet it barely mentions corned beef. Its popular association with boiled cabbage and nationality Diner dismisses as a latter-day development, something deliberately created in the 1920s and 1930s. This was when, writes Diner, "Irish Americans began to experiment a bit with the presentation of identity through food."[51] Prior to that, so traumatized were they by the Great Famine that food carried no meaning as far as Irishness was concerned. Diner does not explain how it came to pass that famine detached food from Irish identity when it clearly failed to do so in the case of the French, a people subjected to famine at least seventy-five times over the past several hundred years.[52] And what about the food-obsessed Chinese, who parse food and identity ever so finely and whose experience with catastrophic starvation has been both frequent and relatively recent?

Historically, the connection between corned beef and Ireland appears to reach back as far as the eleventh century. Alan Davidson writes that much of its history has been that of a holiday dish.[53] Easter Sunday, the most important festival of the year in Ireland, occasioned feasting on lamb, veal, and chicken, but the meal people took greatest pleasure from was corned beef accompanied by cabbage and floury potatoes.[54] Refugees from the Great Famine carried this tradition with them to America, where they promptly transferred it to Saint Patrick's Day. The city of Cork produced immense quantities of corned beef for export from the late seventeenth to the early nineteenth century. Much of it was shipped to Great Britain and continental Europe. However, judging from the early dietaries, no other nationality favored corned beef nearly as much as the Irish. Indeed, among no other people studied by nineteenth-century nutritionists did corned beef show up in even a quarter of the households sampled.

Was the singular importance of corned beef in the Irish American diet an artifact of economy rather than identity? In other words, was it merely a matter of sorely impoverished immigrants purchasing an especially cheap meat? Not likely. The early dietaries show that Irish immigrants spent an average of twenty-two cents per day on food, considerably more than most of their counterparts. Bohemians, particularly those new to the United States, fed themselves for much less (just sixteen cents per day) and without any help from corned beef.[55] The only other late nineteenth- and early twentieth-century immigrant homes in which corned beef maintained at least a peripheral presence were British, French Canadian, and German. Of these, the Germans typically ate more cheaply than the Irish.[56] The British and French Canadian diets stood out as two of the most expensive.[57]

How can we explain the challenges to corned beef's history as an important Irish food? Why do some Americans of Irish ancestry snipe at its place on the Saint Patrick's Day table and belittle its presence as inauthentic? The main reason, it would appear, arises from the feeling that corned beef usurped the historical place of bacon, and, in fact, those who decry all the fuss about eating corned beef on Saint Patrick's Day usually champion bacon as the more genuinely Irish meat for festive occasions. And, indeed, such was the case; historically, the only meat available to Ireland's poor was bacon, and there is no question that it was the star of many, and very likely most, tables on holidays and holy days back in Ireland. Food writer Bridget Haggerty recalled that when she was growing up, her dad brought home a nice piece of boiled bacon, a meat more like ham than American bacon.[58] Her mother boiled potatoes in the jacket and occasionally served cabbage to accompany it, with soda bread and plenty of butter on the side. Corned-beef feasting, by Haggerty's reckoning, originated with nostalgic Irishmen living abroad who tried to create a meal that would remind them of home. The reason they did not accompany their recollections with bacon processed in the Irish manner was because cured pork was not what people aspired to eat. When Irish immigrants could afford a proper festive meal come Saint Patrick's Day, there was no convincing them to eat bacon. Been there, done that, as the saying goes. Corned beef was what proper folks ate; bacon was for those who could afford no better. A person in America might not be wealthy, but he or she could eat like a gentleman or lady did back in Ireland. And if corned beef was good for the holidays, why not every Sunday—indeed, why not two or three or more days every week?

Corned beef, of course, was not the only distinctive food in the Irish American diet. The bacon just mentioned also was a primary core commodity and not particularly popular among other European immigrants. Mutton, condensed milk, barley, wheat rolls, fruit pies, and soda crackers were characteristic secondary foods. Peripheral items not found in the typical European American pantry included dried beef, beef tripe, lamb, salt cod, dairy cream, doughnuts, buns, dried and canned peas, corn starch, and sauerkraut.

The Irish American diet tended to be energy rich. Nutritionally, it resembled the Bohemian diet, with animal products providing close to 45 percent of its fuel value (see table 5.2). Compared to Bohemians, however, Irish immigrants took in even more fat. At the same time, they consumed considerably less protein. This can be traced in large part to a robust appetite for fatty meats. That appetite, however, diminished remarkably among second-generation Irish Americans.[59]

British Americans

The wholesale emigration of British peoples out of England, Scotland, and Wales began early in the nineteenth century. Substantial numbers arrived in the United States prior to midcentury. The influx gathered steam in the 1860s.

Immigration from Great Britain rose for the next several years, subsided briefly, and then increased again, bringing a mixture of well-educated professionals, skilled craftsmen, and unskilled laborers to American shores. This ended with the financial panic of 1893, but during the prior decade an average of more than eighty thousand people a year emigrated from Great Britain to the United States.[60]

Between 1893 and 1897, researchers collected five dietaries from households of British immigrants.[61] Three of them—two in Chicago, one in New York—appeared to be prosperous. The other two, both in Pittsburgh, subsisted in a sorry state.[62]

Kingsley House, a Pittsburgh settlement project, nominated the two Pittsburgh households for study. Isabel Bevier, who came over from the Pennsylvania College for Women (today's Chatham College) to work with Kingsley House, led the inquiry. In one household, she found three sickly children. The family was trying to survive the winter on little more than stale bread, butterine, and lard. The blacksmith who headed the household appeared thin and delicate. He suffered from a lung disease that prevented him from working. Members of the other household, barely surviving on a meager income and hounded by creditors, became convinced that Bevier's investigation was part of a scheme to reduce wages. They ended their participation eight days into an intended month-long study. Bevier, reviewing materials collected up to that point, felt that the homemaker in this case had grossly overstated her food purchases from the start. These data were not used to calculate average intakes.

Nevertheless, the averages listed for British Americans in table 5.2 tended to be high. The fuel value of the food consumed in one household amounted to over 5,000 Cal/m/d, with a mean of 3,800 Cal/m/d for all of the households. This surpassed the overall average for European immigrants by nearly 13 percent. It exceeded Old World estimates by even more, topping an average for Scottish workers in Edinburgh by 17 percent.[63] It topped the average energy intake for a representative set of impoverished households in York, England, by roughly 30 percent.[64]

Still, British immigrants ate more or less the same kinds of victuals as their counterparts in Great Britain. The inventories, in fact, specify a diet very much along the lines of the typical Irish American pattern described previously. The only major departures were the addition of pigs' feet as a core dietary product and the demotion of corned beef and cabbage to peripheral status.

In addition to eating much the same foods as people ate in Great Britain, British immigrants divided their food budgets between animal and vegetable products in nearly the same proportions. They got much more for their money in the United States, however, particularly when it came to meat and dairy products. These foods probably contributed about 30 percent of the energy consumed by Edinburgh's working class.[65] By comparison, commodities from animal sources supplied an average of more than 40 percent of the food energy consumed in British American households (see table 5.1). Fat accounted for most of the difference. Animal fat contributed an average of 32 percent of the energy contained in immigrant diets (see table 5.1). This compared with an average donation of approximately 20 percent to the working-class diets documented in Edinburgh.[66] Remarkable differences existed as well with respect to protein intakes. Members of poor working-class families in York consumed just short of 90 g/m/d of protein from all sources.[67] A sample of fifteen working-class families in Edinburgh returned an average of nearly 100 g/m/d from all sources and just over 40 g/m/d from animal products.[68] British immigrants to the United States exceeded these intakes by far, consuming, on average, 78 g/m/d of protein from animal sources and 133 g/m/d from animal and vegetable sources combined (see table 5.2).

German Americans

Between 1840 and 1880, the majority of America's new arrivals came from the German states.[69] Among these newcomers were a relatively small number of well-educated political refugees, but for the most part the immigrants were peasant farmers who faced grim prospects at home.[70] Once in the United States, about half of them remained committed to an agrarian way of life. Many of the others headed directly to cities. Baltimore, New York City, and Philadelphia attracted large German-speaking populations, but proportionally German immigration had a greater effect on cities further west. Cincinnati, Cleveland, and Milwaukee were over 40 percent German by 1900. Omaha became nearly 60 percent German American.[71]

Eighteen dietaries recorded food consumption among the German immigrants of the Gilded Age. Richards and Shapleigh produced five studies in

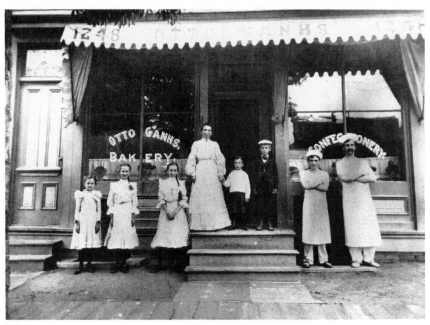

PHOTO 5.3
"Remember When . . . Bakery Smells Filled the Neighborhood?" (1902). Immigrant Otto
Granhs and his family supplied their German-speaking Milwaukee neighborhood with
bread, doughnuts, cakes, and confections. (Photograph by *Milwaukee Journal.* Courtesy
of Remember When [RW1017], Historic Photo Archives, Milwaukee Public Library.)

Philadelphia during the winter of 1892 and three more in Chicago the following
spring.[72] The OES's New York series contained ten studies, six describing what
families ate during the spring and three listing foods consumed in late summer.[73]
All of the households recruited for these investigations lived in depressed neighborhoods, and some of the families were exceptionally poor. In one instance, a
woman whose husband had sustained brain damage at work was attempting to
support him and their five children by making dresses. Other women cooked,
did laundry, sold newspapers, or kept a small shop in order to help feed their
families. Most, however, were full-time homemakers. Several of their husbands
worked as carpenters. Other occupations included boarding house proprietor,
fish peddler, jeweler, longshoreman, and restaurant carver.

The typical diet of a German immigrant household conformed closely to
the standard Euro-American model (see table 5.1). Wheat bread and pota-

toes provided the bulk of the diet along with a number of secondary items, including wheat rolls, rye bread, cake, rice, and beans. German Americans consumed animal products to a lesser extent than the Bohemian, British, and Irish immigrants, but, nonetheless, fresh beef, pork, eggs, and milk occupied central places on the table. Round steaks and shoulder roasts rated as favorite cuts of beef. Chops ranked far and away as the most popular cut of pork. In the dairy category, German families shared with the Irish a taste for condensed milk. It rated as a secondary core victual along with aged cheese. Fieldworkers referred specifically to one such cheese, Limburger, by name.

When it came to fresh vegetables and fruits, German Americans placed the tomato, whether fresh or canned, at the very center of their diet alongside the onion and cabbage. Sauerkraut occupied a secondary place on the annual menu because of the superior appeal of fresh spring and summer greens. Red cabbage, a peripheral food, did not appear in the dietaries of other immigrant nationalities.

German immigrants ate cheaply. Budget data for eight ethnic groups in New York City reveal that across all income brackets, on average only African Americans spent a smaller proportion of their income on food.[74] Dietaries indicated that only Orthodox Jews and recently arrived Bohemians spent less money on food than Germans. Thus, it comes as no surprise that average energy consumption among German immigrants was relatively low. At just over 3,000 Cal/m/d (see table 5.2), their energy consumption was roughly the same as the average for blacks living in the poorest areas of New York City and Philadelphia.

The parsimony of German immigrants may have been as much a matter of habit as economic necessity. This suggestion arises from an 1885 study of impoverished German handweavers in Zittau, Saxony.[75] The project produced eleven dietaries in a region where impoverished agricultural and industrial workers took in an average of just 2,290 Cal/m/d.[76] Zittau's weavers ate the typical "potato diet" of the region. Actually, "potato diet" was a misnomer. More than half of the food consumed consisted of bread. This was precisely the kind of fare that many immigrants were accustomed to before they left Germany. It provided the handweavers and their families with an average of 2,594 Cal/m/d. Their diet typically offered milk and butter daily, except in the midst of winter, but only on Sunday did it contain a little meat.[77]

Consistent with this pattern, the typical diet of a German American immigrant contained a liberal allowance of dairy products and was relatively rich in animal carbohydrates. But protein intake, especially animal protein, was low by American standards (see table 5.2). In contrast, the consumption of animal fat was copious. It contributed about 30 percent of energy intake. Total fat contributed only slightly less energy to the diets of German immigrants as it did to the diets of British, Irish, and Italian immigrants. Nevertheless, the average fat intake of German Americans represented a huge boost over the level of fat consumption recorded among working-class Germans. The Zittau weavers, for example, acquired, on average, a mere 16 percent of their food energy in the form of fat. Bavarian brewery workers, taking in almost 4,400 Cal/m/d, drew an average of only 13 percent of their energy from fat.[78]

The corpus of German American dietaries includes five studies conducted in the homes of American-born families. These second-generation German Americans, all Chicagoans, were poverty stricken. They nevertheless managed to spend, on average, roughly two cents more a day per person for food than their immigrant counterparts. This, however, did not translate to meatier and leaner diets. As among the Bohemians, average intakes of animal fat and carbohydrates from nonanimal sources climbed. Protein intake from animal sources remained about the same. Average energy consumption increased in second-generation households, though not nearly as much as among Bohemians who had lived in the United States for many years.

EATING LIKE KINGS

Many newcomers to the United States, even those in very meager circumstances, felt they were eating like kings. Conditions may have been far from rosy, but, generally speaking, they were immensely better than those endured in Europe. Werner Sombart, writing about the failure of socialism to gain much ground in America, explained how difficult it was to convince people that they were downtrodden when every day they had four times as much bread and potatoes and three times as much sugar as German laborers.[79]

The nutritional differences from one side of the Atlantic to the other were as impressive as Sombart's multipliers imply. A comparison of American and European dietaries indicates that immigrants routinely consumed 10–15 percent more food energy than their former countrymen. The American ad-

vantage amounted to over 35 percent in some cases. From a nutritional standpoint, an unskilled and nearly penniless German laborer effectively moved up
the class ladder by relocating to America. His family, once settled in Chicago
or New York, could reasonably expect to sit down to three meals a day as rich
in energy as the repasts that skilled mechanics in Munich ate regularly.[80] Even
a German professional, estimated to consume an average of 2,565 Cal/m/d,
could anticipate a substantial boost in energy intake upon immigrating to the
United States, where the middle-class average appears to have exceeded 3,000
Cal/m/d (see table 4.3).

The principal reason for the substantial difference in the energy content
of American and European diets had to do with fat. Foods containing ample
amounts of fat were abundant and cheap in America compared to the other
side of the Atlantic, and moving to the United States normally entailed big
increases in fat consumption. For example, dietaries taken in the homes of
British immigrants indicated an average consumption of total fat amount-
ing to three and a half times the average calculated for poor working-class
families in Great Britain.[81] Meals taken in the homes of British immigrants
included, on average, almost twice the fat contained in the rations of Her
Majesty's Royal Engineers.[82] The picture apparently was much the same for
immigrants from Eastern and Central Europe. Investigators found an average fat intake among Chicago's Orthodox Jews to be more than two and a
half times greater than an average for peasants living in the Moscow area.[83]
Similarly, studies revealed that the diet of German immigrants in the United
States contained over two and a half times as much fat as the diet of Germans who remained at home. The diet of German Americans with little by
way of financial resources contained about 10 percent more fat than the diet
of professionals residing in Germany.[84]

As with fat, so with protein. The average intake recorded among British
immigrants topped an estimate for Great Britain's working-class poor by
around 70 percent.[85] Average protein consumption among German American immigrants amounted to more than one and a half times that documented for members of Germany's working-class poor.[86] Differences of such
magnitude help explain why the average American-born male stood 2.1 cen-
timeters (0.84 inches) taller than the average European-born male residing
in the United States.[87] Even greater were the differences in average stature

between Americans and their cousins who remained on the other side of the Atlantic. These can be attributed to the same processes discussed in the previous chapter. Just as members of America's privileged classes, because of their superior diets, came closer to meeting their genetic potential for growth than members of America's working class, so, too, those youngsters who grew up in the United States had the advantage over those who grew up in Europe. The higher protein contents (and fuel values) of American diets facilitated achieving full stature by reducing the likelihood of episodic and irremediable interruptions in growth.[88]

Nutritional balance was another issue. Here there was remarkable disparity among immigrant nationalities. Table 5.4 illustrates this by comparing immigrants in terms of the variety of foods typically included in their diets. Data pertaining to a Chinese household located in San Francisco and French

Table 5.4. Average Cost and Dietary Variety among Twelve Sets of Immigrants

NATIONALITY	FOODS / WEEK		Average Cost ($/m/d)
	7-Day Average	14-Day Average	
Chinese		20	0.19
American-born Bohemians	29		0.34
French Canadians (Chicago)		18	0.23
American-born Germans	27		0.21
Bohemians (in US >10 years)	25	15	0.19
Russian Orthodox Jews		15	0.18
Irish	23		0.22
Russian Liberal Jews	20	13	0.22
Bohemians (in US <10 years)	20	12	0.16
Germans	19		0.19
British	18		0.26
Italians	18		0.23

Canadian families in Chicago come up for discussion in the next chapter, but they are included in order to facilitate comparisons. The average number of different food items consumed over the course of seven or fourteen days serves to indicate the extent of dietary variety. The table supplies some economic context by reporting the average cost of groceries for each set of immigrants listed.

The tabulations make two things clear: first, that there existed great disparities among ethnic diets from the standpoint of variety, and second, that variety from one nationality to the next did not depend entirely on the amount of money spent at the food store. The table's seven-day averages range from twenty-nine different foods for native-born Bohemian Americans to eighteen distinct items for both British and Italian immigrants. The fourteen-day averages top out at twenty items per week in Chinese kitchens and drop down to just twelve items per week for Bohemians who had been settled in the United States for less than ten years. American-born Bohemians and foreign-born Chinese Americans had diets almost equally varied. Yet they spent vastly different sums for the foods they ate. The same can be seen at the other end of the spectrum with German, British, and Italian immigrants all purchasing less than twenty different foods per week on average. Variety was about the same, but British families paid around seven cents per man per day more for groceries than the Germans and about three cents per man per day more than the Italians.[89]

These disconnects can be explained in part as cultural happenstance. Every immigrant group came to America with their tastes well defined in advance. The Chinese had the good fortune of finding their tastes, broad as they were, cheaply satisfied in the United States. The Italians, as noted earlier, were not so lucky. Given their poverty and the high cost of many of the foods they loved, folks from Italy had to content themselves with fewer commodities than they might have otherwise.

This may have been the case for Bohemians and Germans as well. However, in their cases, there exists data to show that variety increased over time. Dietaries collect from German Americans indicate a gap from first- to second-generation households of eight additional foods per week, purchased at an extra cost of around two cents per man per day. Table 5.4 relates basically the same story for Bohemians. Furthermore, it shows that Bohemians who had

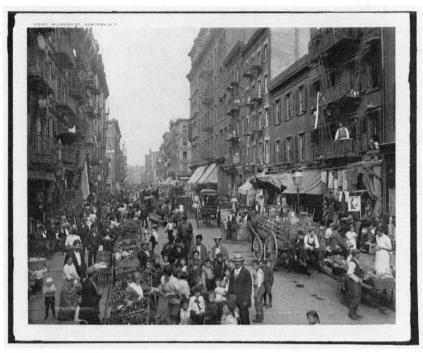

PHOTO 5.4

"Mulberry St., New York, NY." (c. 1900). Italians dominated this street market and the surrounding area after displacing previous sets of earlier immigrants, including British, German, and Irish. (Courtesy of the Detroit Publishing Company Photograph Collection [LC-DIG-det-4a08193], U.S. Library of Congress, Prints and Photographs Division.)

lived in the United States for more than ten years spent about five cents per man per day more on food than those who had lived in the United States for less than ten years. That extra five cents apparently enabled families to add an additional three to five foods to their weekly shopping baskets.[90]

THE NUTRITIONAL CONSEQUENCES

Although Gabaccia finds the late nineteenth century to be a time of culinary conservatism, clearly it produced radical changes in nutrition, especially among immigrants and their children. This may seem paradoxical, but there is no logical reason why such sweeping nutritional amendments could not occur in an essentially conventional milieu.

The key to understanding what took place is to appreciate that the culinary conservatism of the immigrant revolved around ideals that remained unrealized in Europe. In America, however, they were realized. The dishes that many had only savored in their thoughts actually began appearing on their plate. Sunday and holiday feasts became everyday fare. Scots, who had taken pleasure in a piece of bacon or a shred of corned beef once a week, ate meat three times a day in places like Chicago and Pittsburgh. Bohemians, whose milk had been stripped of cream in Czechia, bought milk with cream in Chicago and drank it year round. St. Louisans from Campania, who once had to be content with watching others eat spaghetti, could now cover it with tomato sauces rich in pig fat or olive oil and delight in it every day. Owing to drastic differences in just about everything else that governed their access to food, Old World tastes in no way inhibited great changes in the quantity and quality of immigrants' nutrition.

These were positive changes for the most part. The added energy, extra protein, and better balance were far from superfluous judging from anthropometric records. But were there downsides? Did the jump from an intake of around 3,400 Cal/m/d for newly immigrated Bohemians to an average of over 4,000 Cal/m/d among American-born Bohemians go beyond the bounds of a healthy nutritional improvement? Immigrant diets contained more protein than before, especially protein from animal sources, but at the same time they were loaded with more animal fat and stripped of complex carbohydrates. Did these shifts lead to the increased risks of heart disease and colon cancer we see today?

Questions like these come to mind because studies of modern immigrants have revealed some serious snags in the American dream. One of these is obesity, a condition in which a person weighs more than 20 percent above what is considered optimum for a specific age, height, and body build.[91] A recent inquiry found obesity to be rare among foreign-born Americans but only so long as they have lived in the United States less than ten years.[92] After ten years, the story is different. By fifteen years, the nation's diet and lifestyle begin to exact a toll, and the obesity rate among immigrants jumps to 19 percent. The percentage at this point stands just three points shy of that for the general population suffering from obesity and all of its medical consequences, including an increased risk for type 2 diabetes, high blood pressure, and death from cardiovascular disease.

There is no telling whether dietary changes among immigrants one hundred years ago affected them in the same way, but it seems unlikely. The reason has little to do the differences in the kinds of food people eat nowadays as opposed

to the kinds that people ate back then. Immigrants at the outset of the twentieth century, no less than those recently arrived, went from diets containing 20
percent or less total fat to diets in which animal fats alone contributed as much
as 40 percent or more to the total energy intake. Newcomers from Europe in
the 1890s, no less than today's Asian immigrants, almost overnight went from
diets consisting primarily of complex vegetable carbohydrates to diets in which
vegetables provided less than 50 percent of the energy. These changes were occurring long before the existence of fast foods—in fact, they were occurring
many years before the development of a fully industrialized food system. This
means that prior to lifestyle advertising, convenience culture, or whatever other
aspect of contemporary life one might wish to blame, immigrants ate like kids in
a candy store. With sharp appetites for nutrients that had been scarce in the Old
World and were now plentiful in the New World, they ate it with little thought of
restraint. If the immigrants of yesteryear and their offspring were not victims of
excess in the same ways that immigrants are today, it very likely was because the
late nineteenth century presented more physically demanding environments.
After all, America was still two world wars, a Great Depression, and many years
of manual labor away from becoming the land of sedentary living that it is today.

Contrasts

Gilded Age dietaries tell of remarkable differences in eating habits from North to South and between East and West. They also expose inconsistencies across gender lines. These become apparent as we turn our attention from household dietaries to those that focused instead on eating clubs, canteens, mess halls, and other sorts of collective dining rooms.

Much of the work of Atwater-era nutritionists was carried out in student boarding facilities. Investigations took place on college campuses in several parts of the country. The results reveal regionalisms that, from the standpoint of household dietaries, are hard to detect. The same goes for gender differences. Although these are rendered invisible by the methodology of household dietaries, they become readily visible in collegiate studies thanks to the sexual segregation of nineteenth-century dining halls. Dietaries conducted among members of sports teams and work groups offer additional opportunities for comparative study. Of particular interest here are research results that allow us to compare the cultures of East and West. We examine these through food inventories recorded among Chinese and French Canadian immigrants and at the athletic training tables of Harvard and Yale, paying special attention to the diets of men engaged in extremely strenuous activities.

COLLEGE EATING CLUBS AND DINING HALLS: REGIONAL PATTERNS
University psychologists, already notorious by 1900 for requiring undergraduates to serve as the subjects of their experiments, had close rivals among

early nutritionists. Between 1893 and 1902, nutritionists published more than fifty dietaries recounting the eating habits of college men and women. Thirty of these inquiries involved individual students at Harvard University.[1] The rest, conducted at a variety of public and private institutions, queried collective food use in campus boarding houses, eating clubs, and dining halls. The belief that what collegians ate at school reflected the eating habits of the communities and social circles from which they came provided justification for many of these studies. This belief made sense because many collegians at the time took their meals as members of private associations called "eating clubs." These are not found on most campuses nowadays, but in their heyday eating clubs existed as student-run voluntary societies organized to relieve individual members of the need to prepare their own meals.

Organization was simple. Club members paid dues and elected one of their own to serve as steward. The steward hired a cook. He also made arrangements for kitchen and dining facilities and, in some instances, did the marketing. At the University of Georgia, a volunteer faculty member served as steward for the Students' Boarding Club, a group that boasted no less than one hundred members.[2] The club elected an oversight committee to work directly with the steward. Members and their parents perpetually concerned themselves with keeping costs down. The university helped by granting the club facilities, including a kitchen, pantry, dining room, and furnishings, all free of charge.

Eating clubs enjoyed a great deal of collective autonomy when it came to menu planning. Large colleges and universities hosted multiple clubs catering to different tastes and budgets. Wesleyan University, for example, had several clubs, among them one for women, another for men steadfastly committed to low-cost board, and yet another determined to provide abundant meals featuring a variety of attractive dishes three times a day.[3] Charles Wait, the chemist involved in nutrition studies at the University of Tennessee, kept track of the diets of three boarding clubs on the university's campus.[4] The smallest, a group associated with the university farm, enrolled just thirteen men, all of them sons of Tennessee farmers. Most of the members earned part of their tuition doing the same barnyard chores for the university that they were accustomed to doing at home. Each member contributed two dollars a week toward the purchase of food and to pay the salaries of the club matron and her assistants. A second group, the College Club, enrolled forty-one men, most of them from rural areas of the state. Members generally came from affluent families, but nonetheless the club dedicated itself to low-budget dining. Finally, there was University Boarding House, a venue with a substantial staff of professionals trained to serve the less cost conscious. A number of professors took their meals at University Boarding House.

Not every institution of higher learning left the matter of feeding students to clubs. Some colleges operated their own facilities. Food usage in institutionally managed dining halls was researched at the University of Chicago; Maine State University (today's University of Maine); Lake Erie College in Painesville, Ohio; and Cleveland's Western Reserve University (now part of Case Western Reserve).[5] Investigators at Chicago and Lake Erie concerned themselves exclusively with the nutrition of college women. Research at Western Reserve took place in both men's and women's dining halls.

Unlike the fast-food model currently emulated by college food services, the ideal college dining facility during the Gilded Age simulated eating at home. At institutions where students generally came from well-to-do homes, this required dining-hall staff to accentuate culinary variety, attentive service, and fine table settings. The University of Chicago offered weekly receptions and other special entertainments as part of residential life.[6] Food costs for female residents came to just over twenty-two cents a day, but the full cost of board came to nearly twice that because of the amenities that attended dining. Guilford House at Western Reserve operated in a similar fashion. The College for Women exercised direct management through a housemistress, but it did not seek to profit from room and board. The principal objective was to provide ample, well-served meals that reminded coeds of home.[7] For Adelbert Hall, a facility boarding sixty-three men, Western Reserve avoided direct management by procuring the services of a matron, an "experienced woman" the school entrusted with providing "an ample and wholesome diet at a moderate cost."[8] She purchased vegetables at the public market, went to the local bakery for bread, and bought meat and eggs wholesale. Her regular boarders paid three dollars per week for their meals.

Even a century ago, college students in various regions of the country were already eating much the same thing. This was especially true comparing the Northeast (as represented in six dietaries) to the Midwest (as represented in seven dietaries).[9] Few foods central to the typical diet of one region were missing from the typical diet of the other. The only core items noted on northeastern menus that failed to show up in the Midwest were beef liver, mutton, salt cod, and oysters. Hominy, a popular food among students in New England, appeared on only one of the midwestern campuses. Another remarkable difference involved the frequent use of cottolene, margarine, and vegetable oils at the midwestern institutions. Lard remained the undisputed king of the cooking fats in the Northeast. Midwestern students often drank skimmed milk. Those in the Northeast did not.

Apart from these few differences, a student transferring from one region to the other would have found nothing unfamiliar on the menu. The core of the diet in both parts of the country consisted of fresh meat, specifically beef, lamb, and pork. Among the beef cuts, students in both regions favored rib and sirloin roasts, as well as porterhouse, round, and sirloin steaks. As for lamb, it was most often the leg. Chops were preferred when it came to pork. Cured pork, particularly bacon and ham, appeared regularly on the menu, as did fresh poultry. Turkey often graced the table on the northeastern campuses. Chicken was served more often in the Midwest. From Connecticut to Missouri, clubs and institutional food services routinely offered Graham bread as an alternative to white bread, presumably to cater to the health conscious. Although Graham flour was used in far smaller quantities than white flour, researchers noted its presence in more than half of the dining rooms sampled in both regions. Hot and cold breakfast cereals, such as Wheatlet and shredded wheat, were popular enough to rank as core foods in New England as well as the Midwest, and in both regions dining halls made heavy use of canned goods, including salmon, corn, tomatoes, and various fruits, especially peaches.

A comparison of the typical collegiate diet of New England and the Midwest with the typical diet of the eating clubs at the Universities of Georgia and Tennessee reveals several substantial differences. To start with, four items core to the typical diet of southern students—buttermilk, sweet potatoes, radishes, and pickles—were peripheral to the diet of northern students.[10] Grits and cowpeas were entirely absent. Conversely, thirteen foods core to the typical diet in the North occupied the peripheries of the collegiate diet in the South. Corned beef, beef liver, pork sausage, and lamb fit into this category, as did bananas, oranges, and prunes.[11] Fourteen foods central to the typical diet of northern students did not appear at all in the inventories collected on southern campuses.[12] Among the missing items were dried beef, bacon, salt cod, oysters, prepared breakfast cereals, and Graham bread.[13]

A look at the nutritional contents of the diets of college men uncovers little difference between the North and South save for relatively high total fat values for the northern diets, especially in the Midwest. At the Universities of Georgia and Tennessee, students took in less animal carbohydrates, fat, and protein than their northern counterparts because clubs allocated less money toward the purchase of meat and dairy products. Such items claimed a bare 52 percent of southern students' food expenditures. They accounted for almost 65 percent of the food dollars spent by eating clubs and institutional food services in the Northeast and Midwest, a percentage not out of line with the domestic budgets of professionals and skilled laborers.

The high fat content of northeastern and midwestern students' diets came from large and frequent servings of beef and pork and large quantities of milk. Milk fat in the diets recorded at Wesleyan and Maine State averaged nearly 75 g/m/d compared to less than 45 g/m/d at Tennessee and Georgia. At Western Reserve, where milk was served ad lib three times a day to male undergraduates, dairy-fat intake averaged 83 g/m/d. At the University of Missouri, situated at the edge of the Ozark Mountains far to the west of Western Reserve, club fare contained relatively little dairy fat.[14] This, coupled with a substantial infusion of pork fat, made the nutritional pattern look, in some respects, more southern than typically northern. Still, there was plenty of beef consumption and a substantial amount of beef fat in the diet. Not counting cottolene, the beef-fat content averaged 33 g/m/d on northeastern campuses and 44 g/m/d on midwestern campuses, more than double the average for the Upland South.[15]

Eating Habits and Gender

Diet and nutrition one hundred years ago varied across gender lines to a remarkable extent. Two sets of data, the first collected by W. O. Atwater and his group at Wesleyan University in Middletown, Connecticut, the second by O. F. Tower at Western Reserve University in Cleveland, Ohio, attested most convincingly to the differences.[16] Both investigations amounted to controlled comparisons, gauging the eating habits of men and women on the same campus at the same point in the school year (April and May).

Tower, unlike the Wesleyan investigators, drew explicit attention to gender differences. He noted big discrepancies in meat consumption. Male students consumed a wider variety of meats and a broader assortment of meat cuts than females. The matron in charge of Adelbert Hall, the men's residence, purchased meat by the side or quarter. The matron in charge of Guilford House, the women's residence, confined her orders to certain retail cuts, primarily beef sirloin roasts and steaks. The women of Guilford House liked cured pork (bacon and ham in particular), but, unlike the men, they did not eat pork chops, loins, ribs, and sausages.

When it came to different sorts of foods, the shoe was on the other foot and women enjoyed the greater variety. Unlike the men, they ate cheese often and used cream every day. Tower registered just fourteen vegetable species other than grains and dried legumes for the men's dining room over a two-week period. Over the same period, the women of Guilford House ate no less than forty-seven vegetable foods, discounting grains and dried legumes. Tower found this difference remarkable, but he offered no good explanation for it. To many, it appeared wasteful. After all, fruits and veg-

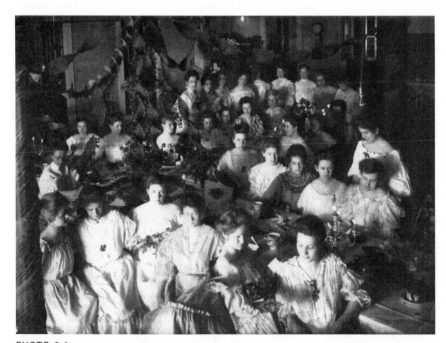

PHOTO 6.1
"Oxford College Dining Room" (c. 1890). Students seated in the festively decorated commons of the former Oxford Female Institute. Here proper eating habits were undoubtedly cultivated. (Photograph by Frank R. Snyder. Courtesy of the Smith Library of Regional History, Oxford, Ohio.)

etables were relatively costly. Yet, as far as chemists could tell at the time, their only purpose was to aid digestion.

The cost of feeding women at Western Reserve was indeed high, though analysis showed that this could not be blamed entirely on vegetable and fruit purchases. Overall, the university spent more than thirty cents per man per day on food for female students and about four and a half cents per day less for males. But only about a penny and a half of this difference came from purchasing additional vegetables and fruits for Guilford House. The remaining three cents went to butchers on account of the relatively expensive cuts of meat usually served in the women's dining room.

Researchers found similar patterns at Wesleyan University and Lake Erie College.[17] At Wesleyan, men again consumed a broad range of meat products while women focused primarily on beef.[18] As at Western Reserve, women did not eat fresh pork or pork sausage. However, over a period of ten days coeds dined on no less than twenty-three fresh and canned vegetables and fruits compared to just sixteen vegetable and fruit dishes made available to male boarders. A ten-day food listing for Lake Erie College contained twenty-five fresh and canned vegetables and fruits. Here the high cost of provisioning elicited administrative concern, but students strongly insisted on being served a dish of fruit daily and especially at breakfast.[19]

The Training Table: Red Meat Barely Cooked

The reason why men were inclined toward meats but showed less interest in vegetables and fruits had to do with athletics and prevailing notions about manhood and nutrition. Success in sports was the measure of the man, and popular opinion held that a key to victory was a diet of lean meat. The notion that eating meat—especially lean red meat barely cooked—improved physical performance was articulated by both dieticians and athletic trainers. Coaches saw to it that the idea was put into practice at the athletes' tables.

Atwater took an early interest in the nutrition of athletes. In 1891, he estimated that the food purchased for the University of Connecticut's football team was sufficient to provide players with about 6,000 Cal/d.[20] Five years later, his colleague Myer Jaffa studied the football team's training table at the University of California.[21] To everyone's astonishment, Jaffa computed net energy consumption at 7,700 Cal/m/d.[22] Perhaps because this number seemed improbably high, Atwater initiated another study of college athletes in the spring of 1898. This time he directed his attention to rowing and enlisted the cooperation of the athletic departments at both Harvard and Yale.[23] They granted Atwater and his staff access to the kitchens and dining rooms that catered to their varsity oarsmen. The research took place on the home campuses of both schools, as well as at facilities in New London, Connecticut, where the two schools met to compete.

The rowers' training tables were set as the experts advised.[24] Their injunction was to feed athletes large helpings of lean meat roasted or broiled but always barely cooked. The menus at Harvard featured beef, lamb, and occasionally mutton. The beef was usually cut from the loin. The lamb and mutton came off the leg. The kitchen trimmed these meats of fat before roasting and serving them rare—not as rare, however, as some of Harvard's other teams preferred. The kitchen also prepared fricasseed chicken, roasted turkey, and broiled fish. The latter was often a breakfast food. Raw, poached, and boiled eggs were frequently on the table as well. At Yale, the trainers preferred their crews to eat beef almost exclusively. The staff occasionally fixed lamb and chicken as a change of pace. Bacon in small amounts appeared with some dishes, but most of it came back to the kitchen uneaten. Fresh pork did not appear on the training tables. This was consistent with the coaches' insistence on lean meats, but it also spoke of the elite status and health consciousness of the student athlete (see below).

Regarding grains and other vegetables, the watchword among athletes was moderation. The only wheat bread served at the training table was supposed to be dried or toasted, and Harvard's kitchen complied. It supplied crews with oatmeal, hominy, shredded wheat, and occasionally corn cakes. Potatoes appeared on the table twice daily, usually baked or mashed with milk and butter. Sometimes boiled rice mixed with a little milk and sugar found its way into the dining room instead of potatoes, and every so often macaroni had a place on the menu. The training table offered a few vegetables (beets, parsnips, green peas, and tomatoes) but no fresh fruits other than oranges, a breakfast standby. Cooked fruits included stewed prunes, rhubarb, and apples. Apple tapioca pudding, custard pudding, or some other pudding containing large amounts of milk and eggs comprised the usual desserts. The crews' coaches prohibited other sweets.

The beverages of choice consisted of milk, water, and beer. The Harvard crews downed large amounts of milk and cream at every meal.[25] Together,

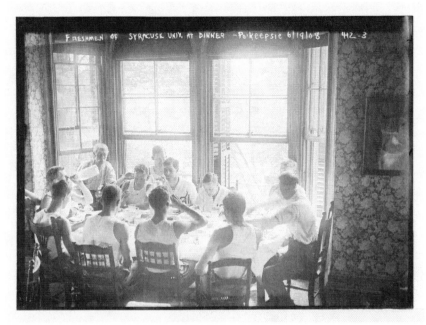

PHOTO 6.2
"Syracuse Freshmen at Dinner, Poughkeepsie" (c. 1908). Members of the university's rowing team and their coaches at the training table. (Photograph by Bain News Service. Courtesy of the George Grantham Bain Collection [LC-USZ62-95949], U.S. Library of Congress, Prints and Photographs Division.)

milk and cream, not to mention substantial helpings of butter and ice cream, supplied the athletes with approximately a quarter of the energy they derived from the animal portion of their diet. The Yale crew, in addition to drinking milk with every meal, drank large quantities of oatmeal water. A staff member made this beverage by adding a small amount of uncooked rolled oats to a pitcher of ice water. The mixture needed to stand for a short time to allow the oats to settle. The particles that floated or remained in suspension were ingested with the water.[26] Beer was a training-table standard. The type preferred at Yale was ale.[27]

Rowing teams' meals delivered plenty of energy but not nearly so much as one might predict based on previous work with football teams. Table 6.1 was prepared to compare selected nutritional values among groups engaged in strenuous activities (see below). It shows that at Harvard and Yale, the oars-

Table 6.1. Average Nutritional Values, Diets Associated with Strenuous Work, 1896–1903

SUBJECTS	ANIMAL CHO (g/m/d)	ANIMAL PROTEIN (g/m/d)	ANIMAL FATS (g/m/d)	% ENERGY ANIMAL
College Rowing Crews	39	114	156	54
Chinese Farm Workers	3	65	90	26
French Canadian Lumberjacks	7	84	338	47
SUBJECTS	VEGETABLE CHO (g/m/d)	TOTAL PROTEIN (g/m/d)	% ENERGY ANIMAL FAT	TOTAL ENERGY (Cal/m/d)
College Rowing Crews	384	157	36	3903
Chinese Farm Workers	676	155	19	4305
French Canadian Lumberjacks	812	187	42	7162

men took in more than 3,900 Cal/m/d. Most of that energy, as the table reveals, came from animal sources. At Harvard, meat and dairy contributed just over 50 percent of the athlete's energy supply. At Yale, they supplied even more. On average, over 40 percent of the energy consumed by the student-athletes came from fats, almost all of them from animal sources. Enormous thirsts for milk and cream contributed considerably to this intake. About one-third of the animal fat consumed at the training table of Harvard's boat crews came from milk and cream. If we include butter and ice cream, dairy fat furnished close to 40 percent of the energy intake derived from animal sources.

How to Be Plump

People in the metropolitan areas of the Northeast and Midwest saw a partiality toward vegetables and fruits and an abstemious attitude toward pork as examples of lady-like deportment. But judging from eating habits at North Dakota Agricultural College (now North Dakota State University), different attitudes prevailed in outlying areas.[28] The women's eating club in Fargo proffered its members just sixteen vegetables and fruits, not counting grains and dried legumes, over a course of twenty days. By comparison, women at the University of Chicago ate forty-one such items that same month over a period of twenty-one days. North Dakota State's coeds dined on pork chops and fresh pork sausages frequently. College ladies further to the east generally did not.[29]

Put simply, upper- and middle-class consumers had come to see pork eating as beneath them. This way of thinking (which pertained specifically to fresh pork, not cured pork) developed in the 1880s with the arrival in eastern markets of fresh beef from the West via the Chicago stockyards. Marketers labeled it "refrigerator beef" and advertised it as a miracle of modern transportation.[30] Promotional campaigns depicted beef eating as fashionable. Pork, by comparison, was unsophisticated; it was old-fashioned country food, a working-class commodity.[31] Polite society permitted it for men, but in some numinous way eating uncured pork degraded the well-bred woman. Besides, even a decade before Upton Sinclair and his exposé, there were questions about cleanliness.[32] People worried about tainted pork. *Good Housekeeping* magazine summed the matter up in 1890, declaring that pork not only failed to win the approval of intelligent people but also was "almost entirely discarded by hygienists" (and sports trainers, too, judging from its absence from training tables).[33]

A century ago, not unlike today, serious concerns existed about the nutritional well-being of fashion-conscious young women. The authors of studies examining the diets of college women appeared sensitive to these, and invariably the researchers commented on their subjects' health. Ellen Richards and Marion Talbot observed, for example, that the new menus tested in the women's residences at the University of Chicago reduced the incidence of headaches.[34] Isabel Bevier and E. C. Sprague noted that students at Lake Erie College appeared to be in excellent health and seemed well satisfied with their diets. The investigators worried, however, that average protein consumption among the women seemed too low.[35] At North Dakota Agricultural College, protein intake was even lower. Edwin Ladd attributed this to eating too little meat.[36] Among the women he studied, nearly half of whom were immigrants, animal flesh added up to about 15 percent of the foods consumed. By comparison, among Wesleyan coeds meat products amounted to roughly one-third of the total food supply. Still, Ladd saw no signs of malnutrition and believed the extent of meat consumption at the ladies' eating club was not out of line by North Dakota standards. The same appeared true regarding the coeds' relatively heavy use of granulated sugar (over 12 percent by weight of total food consumed).

Tower, who found women's protein consumption low at Western Reserve compared to men but generally higher than the average for college students, had another concern.[37] He calculated the energy content of the food served to women to be about the same as the men's. However, to achieve this parity, women consumed disproportionately large quantities of fats. These came chiefly from butter and cream. Tower found, too, that women boarders wasted less food than men. Looking at fat specifically, he discovered the biggest difference. Men threw away upward of 16 percent of the fat on their plates. Women disposed of around 10 percent. The discrepancy was nearly identical at Wesleyan University.[38]

Young ladies' fondness for fat stemmed from essentially the same anxieties that cause many women today to recoil at the thought of eating it. Whether a coed from a wealthy family or a shop girl in less fortunate circumstances, young women aspired to a popular image of loveliness. It called for a certain "florid plumpness," a model of good looks about as far from today's hard, lean look as one can imagine. During the Gilded Age, a slim woman longed to become fleshier. Entertainer Lillian Russell personified the reigning standard of beauty. Her lush body proclaimed health and wealth. A thin body represented disease and destitution. This was why an up-and-coming institution of higher learning like the University of Chicago was pleased to have it known that the meals it served to female residents helped nearly all of them to gain weight over the course of the school year.[39]

For the girl who had to manage her own diet and who felt she needed some advice, there was *How to Be Plump*, a self-help book authored by Chicago physician and homeopath T. C. Duncan.[40] His disquisition, published in 1878, reflected opinions widely held by medical experts.[41] It began by equating thinness with various morbid conditions and a generally unpleasant disposition. Duncan's advice to the young woman unhappy with her slender body was to eat right. That meant having a plain but substantial breakfast of potatoes, meat, fried mush, oatmeal, bread, butter, and well-milked tea or coffee. A hearty dinner was to follow no more than five hours later. The doctor advised that it begin with a proper first course consisting of a light soup, not highly seasoned. The main course was to be built around plenty of vegetables but, again, light use of spices and no condiments. Drinking water with the meal was a bad practice; better for the woman desirous of a voluptuous figure to take chocolate or milk instead. Only in the evening did Duncan permit a dainty meal. He felt that bread and milk or oatmeal and milk were too substantial at this time of day because they might interfere with sleep.

Campus dietaries suggest that Dr. Duncan's precepts were not at all out of tune with practice. Eating clubs and other dining facilities presented female students with approximately 25 percent more food items than they offered males. Vegetables and fruits, the species prescribed for weight gain, made up most of the surplus. College women ate, on average, only half the animal products by weight that men consumed. Even so, women took in only a little less animal fat and 90 percent of the total fat that the average male consumed. Students accomplished this by consuming relatively large quantities of butter, cottolene, cream, eggs, and lard. Western Reserve's coeds, for example, used more butter, lard, and cottolene than their male counterparts. Cream in the women's dining room disappeared at a rate of 56 g/m/d, seven times the average rate in the men's facility. Wesleyan women ate 40 percent more eggs than the university's men. The men used more butter than the women, but the women more than made up the difference by using cottolene at the table in addition to butter. All of this suggests a determination to put on the equivalent of that "freshman fifteen" that twentieth-century college women strive mightily to keep off.[42]

FOOD CULTURES EAST AND WEST

First-generation nutritionists documented food consumption among two sets of non-European immigrants—Chinese and French Canadian. Their diets could hardly have been more dissimilar. However, in the course of recording eating habits among both nationalities, investigators spent time with groups of men engaged in extremely strenuous occupations and in need of fortifying themselves with meals packing immense amounts of energy. The data collected in these instances offer a cross-cultural look at the different ways in which East and West addressed this need and provided men with the required nourishment.

Chinese Americans

Myer Jaffa, assistant professor of agriculture at the University of California, Berkeley, began his work with the conviction that human nutritional needs would never be properly understood by studying central tendencies alone. Computing averages took one only so far; scientists also needed to look at the extremes. Jaffa took his dietary research in that direction by studying eating habits under regimes of intense exertion and deprivation. As mentioned earlier in the chapter, he studied the diet of his university's football team in order to determine the effects of heavy exercise.[43] He documented and analyzed the diet of fruitarians, residents of the Berkeley area who denied themselves any sustenance other than uncooked fruits and nuts.[44] Chinese Americans captured his interest because he and many others believed that they ate little or nothing other than rice. Knowing that many Californians at the time, perhaps no less than today, were intrigued by the idea of a meatless diet, Jaffa saw an excellent opportunity to advance science and at the same time apply the nascent field of nutrition to an issue of popular concern.[45]

With the help of a colleague in the university Department of Oriental Languages, Jaffa and his students conducted three studies.[46] The first recorded eating habits in a situation of light work. The second and third looked at food consumption under separate regimes of moderate and severe work. Jaffa represented diet in an environment of light work by documenting the meals taken by a San Francisco dentist, a Chinese American, and his household. It consisted of the dentist and his wife and seven unrelated men, six of them student boarders, the seventh a resident cook. Jaffa captured a diet addressing moderate work by observing a group of ten laundrymen. All of them lived in the same building in which they worked—a large, one-story wooden structure located in the heart of San Francisco. The men ate and slept together in the main laundry room, bunking under the ironing tables at night. An apprentice hired by the group cooked its meals. To study food consumption under conditions of severe work, Jaffa turned to a gang of twelve men employed to cultivate a forty-five-acre truck farm near Berkeley. Their work day began at six in the morning. It lasted until seven in the evening, with one hour off for dinner. The farm's proprietor housed the men in a shanty attached to his barn. Gang members paid for their board but at a rate below cost in order to compensate for their substandard pay.

Jaffa's three dietaries describe a typical diet consisting of forty foods. Many of these, however, were inventoried only in the household of the San Francisco dentist. Table 6.1 includes data pertaining to his household. It shows values broadly consistent with the other sets of immigrants represented with one obvious exception—a relatively sparse intake of animal-sourced carbohydrates. As these are supplied, for the most part, by milk and dairy products, the scant value can be explained as a consequence of the general distaste for milk typical of Chinese populations.

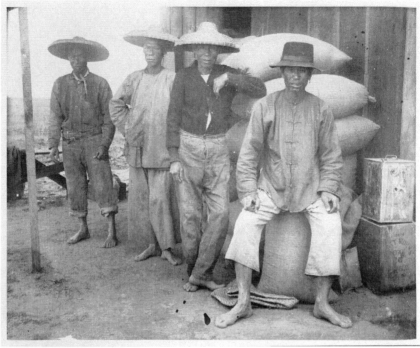

PHOTO 6.3
"Chinese Field Hands, 1898." These laborers probably worked in the Los Angeles area, where photographer C. C. Pierce conducted business. (Photograph by C. C. Pierce. Courtesy of the Photo Archives [photCL Pierce 09878], Huntington Library, Art Collections, and Botanical Gardens.)

The diets of the laundry and farm workers rested on the same foundations as the dentist's: rice, noodles (referred to as "vermicelli" by Jaffa), and bean cheese (possibly fermented bean curd or tofu) comprised the principal foods.[47] The laundrymen also consumed wheat bread and yams in considerable quantities.[48] Provisions consumed in lesser quantities included bean sprouts, green peas, and Chinese cabbage. Other popular items consisted of onions, various radishes, arrowhead tubers, water lily roots, yam bean roots, mustard plants, dried fungus, dried lily flowers, algae, and water chestnuts. Workers on the Berkeley truck farm answered to their many hours of intense labor with a daily ration of rice averaging over 800 g/m/d (close to 2 lb./m/d). Cabbage consumption averaged 230 g/m/d (over 0.5 lb./m/d).[49]

Beef (mainly cut from the round), pork, chicken, and seafood appeared in all three dietaries. The farm workers consumed pork at a rate of just over 200 g/m/d (about 7 oz./m/d). The laundry workers took in a combined total of beef and pork averaging around 300 g/m/d (10.5 oz./m/d). They ate chicken and fish in much smaller quantities, along with some eggs, milk, and butter. The latter three items were not part of the truck-farm diet.

Nutritionally, the farm workers' diet was remarkable. Its energy content averaged more than 4,300 Cal/m/d. Yet only around 25 percent of those calories came from meat and other animal sources. Less than 20 percent derived from any form of fat. Among the European immigrants represented in table 5.1, the contribution of animal fat alone to the energy supply typically exceeded 30 percent while energy from animal sources generally ranged from 40 to 45 percent.

French Canadian Americans

The diet of French Canadian lumberjacks in Maine was an amplified version of the diet of ordinary French Canadian immigrants. Their approach to nutrition, particularly with respect to energy intake, basically turned the Chinese method upside down.

Atwater began studying the food consumption of French Canadians at the behest of the Massachusetts Bureau of Statistics of Labor. In 1885, it responded to public concerns about the living conditions among the state's industrial workers and initiated an inquiry.[50] The investigation included French Canadians, who had been coming to Massachusetts in search of work for many years. The bureau studied representative families and boarding houses. It paid close attention to their food-purchasing habits in East Cambridge, Holyoke, Lawrence, Lowell, and Worcester. Agents traveled to the Canadian province of Quebec and pulled together additional data.[51] This information was turned over to Atwater. He and an assistant analyzed foods similar to those described in the bureau's documents and then used the results to estimate the nutritional contents of local diets.[52]

Later inquiries in Chicago helped develop a more exact picture. Dietaries involving French Canadian immigrants were conducted on the West Side in 1893 and 1895.[53] Investigators encountered a remarkable variety of foodstuffs, indicating considerable dietary diversity. We see this reflected in table 5.3, where French Canadian Americans rate near the top, not far behind Chinese Americans regarding the number of foods typically found in their kitchens.

Otherwise, French Canadians ate like most European immigrants. Keen appetites for salt pork, ham, and pork sausage were distinctive, however. Salt pork was barely seen in the homes of other immigrants. Some granted ham and pork sausage secondary or peripheral places on the table, but Quebecois made both primary foods. Cakes, pies, and cookies qualified as primary core products as well. Pigs' feet, a food beloved by British Americans but not often seen among other immigrants, occupied the secondary core of the typical French Canadian diet.[54]

Immigrants from Quebec not only ate a lot of different foods but also ate a lot—period. In Massachusetts, they consumed, on average, approximately two kilograms (nearly five pounds) of food per day.[55] This was well above average for immigrants at the time, and well above the average for native residents of Quebec.[56] But immigrants could afford it; French Canadians ordinarily earned a great deal more money in the United States than they had back home, and evidently food was a priority, especially meat and dairy items. Massachusetts immigrants consumed over 55 percent more meat and dairy by weight than the average for Quebec. Total food consumption in Chicago was very close to the Quebec average, but in spite of this immigrant families consumed over 60 percent more meat and dairy products by weight than their counterparts in Canada.

For immigrants, more meat and dairy meant diets richer in both animal protein and fat. The cross-border difference in animal-protein consumption was considerable.[57] However, this discrepancy was offset to a large extent among folks who remained in Canada by their greater intake of vegetable protein, much of it from beans. There was, however, no offset in the fat column. The consumption of total fat in Massachusetts nearly doubled that of Quebec, and the intake of animal fat in particular was more than doubled.[58] Over 40 percent of immigrants' energy came from fats in both Massachusetts and Chicago. Fats from animals accounted for 37 percent of the fuel value of French Canadian diets in Chicago (see table 5.3). No other immigrant group came close to the French Canadian's dependence on fats as sources of energy.

C. D. Woods and E. R. Mansfield of the Maine Agricultural Experiment Station discovered that dietary fat provided much of the fuel that French Canadian lumberjacks depended on to harvest the state's timber.[59] The two chemists began studying the diet and nutrition of men employed by the woodcutting industry in the winter of 1901–1902 and continued it the following year. All told, they conducted five separate studies at various locations for periods of up to sixteen days. Their study populations ranged from thirty to fifty men, most of them between twenty-five and thirty years old.

Maine's lumberjacks or loggers were considered a wild bunch. In the popular imagination, their life was one of drinking sprees and hijinks from the moment they broke camp in the spring until they returned to work the following autumn. In camp, however, the men were sober and hardworking. They rose from their cots at five in the morning every day except Sunday. Their work continued with few respites from dawn to dark, and most of them were in bed by nine o'clock.

Logging camps were typically located far from the nearest town. Normally they contained a variety of structures, including an overseer's office, several stables, a blacksmith's shop, and a kitchen or "bean hole." The work crews lived in a large log cabin called "the main camp." It was divided into three sections: the "men's camp," a sleeping area furnished with rough deacon chairs and bunks stacked two high; the "dingle," a lean-to for storing bulky commodities; and the "cookroom." During the fall and winter, while trees were being felled and logs stacked in nearby yards, both cooking and eating took place in the cookroom. It contained bunks for the cook and his assistants, the "cookees." In addition, it housed the furnishings, stoves, utensils, and other accoutrements needed to prepare and dish out meals.

The loggers gathered in the cookroom to eat twice a day, first at 5:15 a.m., then again at 5:30 p.m. Their meals were set out on a table constructed of poles and boards salvaged from old packing boxes. The men sat on benches made of split logs with stakes for legs. As they ate, lumberjacks observed a rule of silence. Harried cooks probably invented this rule to clear the cookroom as soon as possible so that preparations for the next meal could get under way.[60]

The cook usually left his bed to begin work at about 3:45 a.m. He built a fire, prepared breakfast, and at 4:45 a.m. called the cookees to work. Fifteen minutes later, they awoke the work crews, and within another fifteen minutes the cookees had breakfast on the table. At midday, they took dinner out to the work sites, often on sleds. In the spring, when it came time to "drive" the logs to the mill, the cook and his assistants followed the lumberjacks downstream. Meals were prepared in tents and carried to whatever points along the way

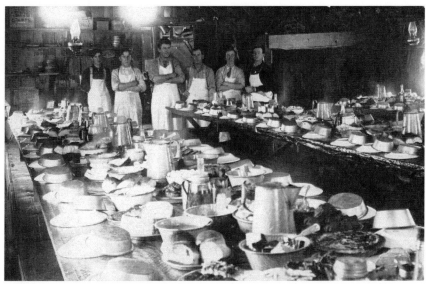

PHOTO 6.4
"Six Cooks Wearing Aprons Stand in a Lumber-Camp Dining Room . . ." (no date). The tables are set for a large encampment of lumbermen in northern Wisconsin. (Courtesy of Albert Greene Heath, collector, Classified File [58394], Wisconsin Historical Society.)

crews happened to be stationed. Because of the grueling work required to keep the drive moving, the loggers needed to eat four or five times a day in order to keep up their strength. Even so, many lost weight.[61]

Lumber-camp meals were always simple and at least twice a day featured baked beans (see table 6.2). The process of preparing meals began in the morning atop an iron stove, where the cook parboiled the beans. In the afternoon, they were carried to the bean hole, a pit several feet deep (a little more than a meter) over which a small cabin was built. The cook's helpers filled the pit with wood to a depth of two feet and set it alight. The fire, once blazing hot, was topped over with stones and pieces of scrap iron. A big pot, filled with alternating layers of the parboiled beans and salt pork, was covered and suspended over the fire pit. When the pot started to boil, the men lowered it directly onto the rocks and iron fragments, which by then were red hot. The pot was then buried in ashes and everything covered over with earth. The next morning, some twelve to fourteen hours later, the cookees dug up the pot for a breakfast of piping-hot beans.

Table 6.2. Typical Menu for the Day, Maine Lumberjacks, Winter 1901–1903

Breakfast	Baked beans, cold meat, biscuits, doughnuts, molasses cookies, stewed prunes, butter, tea, sugar
Dinner	Baked beans, cold meat, biscuits, mashed potatoes, mashed turnips, sugar cookies, stewed prunes, butter, tea, sugar
Supper	Boiled mackerel, cold meat, boiled potatoes, biscuit, loaf bread, butter, sugar cookies, stewed prunes, strawberry jelly, tea, sugar

Dishes prepared in addition to baked beans varied by season. During the winter months, the sourdough biscuit was a mainstay. Cooks worked with fresh forequarters of beef, corned beef (flank and canned), bologna, fresh and salt fish (cod, mackerel, and salmon), condensed milk, lard compound, granulated sugar, and molasses. Other primary foodstuffs consisted of potatoes, onions, turnips, and fruit jellies (currant and strawberry). Smoked pork shoulder, cornmeal, oatmeal, rice, carrots, cabbage, and prunes filled out the secondary core of the typical diet with beef tripe, pork sausage, minced meat, eggs, and syrup among the peripheral commodities.[62]

A proclivity for animal fat; a taste for multiple sweeteners, including refined sugar, molasses, syrups, and fruit jellies; plus hearty appetites for cakes, pies, and cookies combined to make the French Canadian immigrants' diet one of the most energy rich in Gilded Age America. These same traits helped pack the meals of lumberjacks with more energy than any other diet on record. This was necessary because no other occupation exacted such extreme physical demands, especially in the winter. The lumber men needed a considerable number of calories just to keep warm, and against that background the act of chopping a tree at the moderate rate of thirty-five strokes per minute consumed ten calories per minute.[63] Average energy values obtained for the five camps studies by Woods and Mansfield ranged from a little over 5,000 to around 8,500 Cal/m/d.[64]

Most of these calories, as shown in table 6.1, came from carbohydrates. Lumbermen judged the worth of their cooks by how well they prepared dishes composed primarily of carbohydrates. A good cook in the woodsmen's eyes fixed outstanding baked beans, baked first-rate breads, and made exceptionally tasty cakes, pies, and cookies. These items proved profoundly gratifying. The carbohydrates, and especially the simple sugars that the beans and baked goods contained, were digested quickly, raising body temperatures against the cold and relieving feelings of fatigue.[65]

PRUNE AND RAISIN PIES

Lumberjacks acquired a reputation for having a sweet tooth. Henry David Thoreau remarked on it in 1846 after he noticed the great quantity of sweet cakes on the tables of public houses in Maine.[1] "When the lumberers come out from the woods," he wrote, "they have a craving for cakes and pies, and such sweet things."[2] That was because companies at the time placed little importance on indulging the appetites of their men. Policies changed, and by end of the century lumbermen were eating their fill of cakes, pies, and cookies, and their cooks were being hired and fired based on their skills as bakers and pastry makers.[3] This new attitude can be attributed to the industrialization of lumbering. As the pace of work increased and energy demands on employees were notched upward, a diet of practically unlimited fuel value made progressively greater economic sense.[4]

Of all the sweets lumber-camp cooks fed their crews, the men loved pies the most. And of all the pies lumber-camp cooks baked for their crews, the men lavished the greatest praise on prune and raisin. As dried fruits rich in energy and possessing excellent keeping qualities, they were perfect for provisioning hard-working gangs isolated deep in the forests. Long after the mechanization of lumbering, the raisin pie remains a standby in small cafés throughout the North's woods. The prune pie is not nearly as popular as it once was, perhaps because it suffers from the prune's notoriety as a laxative. Nevertheless, as one New England camp cook pronounced, "I'll take the prune. It makes even better apple pie than the peach."[5]

Prune Pie: Use your own pie dough to make this old-time prune pie according to Fannie Farmer's 1896 recipe.[6] It called for half a pound of prunes, half a scant cup of sugar, one tablespoon

(*continued*)

RECIPE 6.1 (*continued*)

of lemon juice, one tablespoon of flour, and one and a half tea-spoons of butter.

Fannie began making her pie by washing and soaking the prunes in a pot containing just enough water to cover them. She then cooked the prunes until soft in the same water. Once the prunes were softened, she removed them from the liquid and took out their pits. Then she cut the pitted prunes into quarters and returned them to the pot with its remaining liquid. She added the sugar and lemon juice. The pot went back on the stove to cook until about one and a half tablespoons of prune liquor remained. By this point, Fannie had ready a pie plate lined with pastry dough. She covered it with the cooked prunes and poured the remaining liquor over them. Fannie dotted this filling with butter and sprinkled it with flour. Finally, she added a top crust and proceeded to bake.

Raisin Pie: The recipe for this filling comes from Maureen Fischer's *Nineteenth-Century Lumber Camp Cooking.*[7] The ingredients consisted of two cups of raisins, one and a half cups of water, a half cup of brown sugar, two tablespoons of all-purpose flour, a half cup of chopped walnuts, and one tablespoon of cider vinegar.

The recipe called for placing the raisins in a pot containing the water, bringing it to a boil, and simmering for five minutes. The brown sugar and flour were then added, and the pot was brought to a boil over medium heat, stirring constantly. The cooking and stirring continued for one minute. The mixture was then removed from the heat, and the chopped walnuts, butter, and vinegar were added. The pot was allowed to cool for ten minutes before the raisin mixture was poured into a pie plate covered with dough. The final steps were to cover the pie with dough for a top crust and to bake it in a 425-degree Fahrenheit oven for twenty-five to thirty-five minutes.

NOTES

1. C. D. Woods and F. R. Mansfield, *Studies of the Food of Maine Lumbermen*, U.S. Department of Agriculture Office of Experiment Stations Bulletin 149 (Washington, DC: U.S. Government Printing Office, 1904), 7.

2. Quoted in ibid., 8.

3. Joseph R. Conlin, "Did You Get Enough Pie? A Social History of Food in Logging Camps," *Journal of Forest History* 23, no. 4 (1979): 182.

4. Ibid.

5. Ibid., 187.

6. Fannie Merritt Farmer, *Boston Cooking-School Cook Book* (Boston: Little, Brown, 1896), 394–95.

7. Maureen M. Fischer, *Nineteenth-Century Lumber Camp Cooking*, Exploring History through Simple Recipes (Mankato, MN: Capstone Press, 2001), 25.

A little less than half of the average energy value of the lumberjacks' diet was consumed in the form of animal products (see table 6.1). Animal fat contributed about 43 percent of the energy intake. As a percentage, total fat did not supply a camp of loggers with much more energy than it supplied to a family of French Canadians in Chicago. Animal fat's contribution to the total energy supply of loggers amounted to only 5 percent more than its contribution to the total energy supply in immigrant households (compare tables 5.1 and 6.1). Thus, the lumberjacks' nutrition remained essentially French Canadian in its proportions while approximately doubling the average fuel values reported for households. This required staggering quantities of food. To feed a camp of one hundred men, a cook at Scott Bog in New Hampshire "daily shoveled out 75 to 100 pounds of beef, a bushel of cookies, 3 bushels of potatoes, 30 pies . . . 21 pound cans of condensed milk, 2 gallons of tinned tomatoes, 3 gallons apples, 16–20 double loaves of bread, and 200 doughnuts. He used 10 yeast cakes a day, 400 pounds of sausage, 25 pounds of liver, 2 gallons of molasses, cabbages in fall and turnips in winter, and tea, coffee, oatmeal, and beans."[66]

Table 6.1 juxtaposes the average values for the three diets that first-generation nutritionists used to gauge the relationship between strenuous activities and diet. Each of the groups involved—Ivy League rowers, Chinese American farmhands, and French Canadian lumberjacks—addressed its nutritional needs from a different direction. Harvard and Yale's boat crews, not unlike the Maasai warriors of Kenya, attacked the matter by filling themselves with milk and blood—or, more accurately, dairy foods and cuts of meat served rare. Of the three, the athletes' diet relied most heavily on animal products to supply energy and protein. It was an expensive diet, with every 150 Cal/m/d costing about one cent.[67] Chinese farm workers, by comparison, relied little on animal sources for their nutrition. Although they consumed nearly as much protein as elite athletes, well over half of it came from grains, legumes, and other vegetable products. Meat and dairy supplied only about a quarter of the farm workers' food energy (see table 6.1). As a result, the men ate inexpensively. Every penny spent added approximate 250 Cal/m/d to the Chinese American farmhand's rice bowl. As for Maine's lumberjacks, they took in somewhat more protein and a lot more carbohydrates than the others (see table 6.1). The lumbermen, unlike the oarsmen, ingested more of their protein from vegetable sources than from animal sources. The same applied for energy; in the lumber camps there was less dependence on foods from animal sources than there was at the athletes' training table.

However, with respect to animal fats specifically, it was another matter. Here the loggers' French Canadian tastes were amply gratified. Plenty of animal fats combined with carbohydrates from such aliments as white flours, dried legumes, refined sugars, and desiccated fruits concentrated a great deal of energy into a relatively small volume of food. This made for an extraordinarily low-cost diet. Every penny spent on provisioning provided workers with approximately 300 Cal/m/d, rendering the lumberjacks' the cheapest of the three high-energy diets studied by the OES researchers. Its economy helps explain why the French Canadian lumberman's diet persisted into the twentieth century and why, in basic outline, it can be considered prototypical of the energy-dense, fast-food formula that remains with us to this very day.

Notes

PREFACE

1. Robert T. Dirks and Nancy Duran, "Agriculture Experiment Station Studies and the History of Food Habits and Nutrition in the United States," *Nutritional Anthropology* 21 (1998): 6–8.

2. Robert T. Dirks and Nancy Duran, "African American Dietary Patterns at the Beginning of the 20th Century," *Journal of Nutrition* 131 (2001): 1881–89.

3. Robert T. Dirks, "Diet and Nutrition in Poor and Minority Communities in the United States 100 Years Ago," *Annual Review of Nutrition* 23 (2003): 81–100.

4. This developed from a paper published as "What Early Dietary Studies of African Americans Tell Us about Soul Foods," *Repast* 26, no. 2 (2010): 8–18.

CHAPTER 1: NUTRITION HISTORY

1. W. O. Atwater, "How Food Nourishes the Body," *Century Illustrated Monthly Magazine* 34, no. 2 (June 1887): 237–52; Atwater, "The Chemistry of Food and Nutrition," *Century Illustrated Monthly Magazine* 34, no. 1 (May 1887): 59–74; Atwater, "The Potential Energy of Food," *Century Illustrated Monthly Magazine* 34, no. 3 (July 1887): 397–405; Atwater, "Pecuniary Economy of Food," *Century Illustrated Monthly Magazine* 35, no. 3 (January 1888): 437–46; Atwater, "Foods and Beverages," *Century Illustrated Monthly Magazine* 36, no. 1 (May 1888): 135–40.

2. K. J. Carpenter, "The Life and Times of W. O. Atwater (1844–1907)," *Journal of Nutrition* 124 (1994): 1707S–14S.

3. Richard Osborn Cummings, *The American and His Food* (Chicago: University of Chicago Press, 1940), 128; Donna R. Gabaccia, *We Are What We Eat: Ethnic Food and the Making of Americans* (Cambridge, MA: Harvard University Press, 1998), 123–24.

4. Archaeologists produce nutrition history by describing food refuse and waste. Their analyses can provide crude but ecologically and sociologically informed impressions of nutrition when they attend to occupational, seasonal, and other differences within extinct communities. Biological anthropologists and their anatomical and osteological studies have done much to uncover nutrition's role in human evolution, but, in addition, they occasionally detect pathologies indicative of nutritional deficiencies in prehistoric and historic skeletal populations. Economic historians have extended their efforts to measure previous generations' standards of living to include biological indicators. Using anthropometrics to gauge nutritional well-being and agricultural production data to represent food supply, economic historians can capture the broad outlines of nutrition history in terms of both inputs and outputs. Nutritionists themselves have not shown great interest in nutrition history, but they do attend to trends and for that purpose keep annual records of nutrient supplies. See Shirley Gerrior, Lisa Bente, and Hazel Hiza, *Nutrient Content of the U.S. Food Supply, 1909–2000*, Home Economics Research Report 56 (Washington, DC: U.S. Department of Agriculture, Center of Nutrition Policy and Promotion, 2004).

5. Ken Albala, "Culinary History," in *Routledge International Handbook of Food Studies*, ed. Ken Albala, 114–21 (London and New York: Routledge, 2013); Barbara Haber, "Culinary History vs. Food History," in *The Oxford Encyclopedia of Food and Drink in America*, ed. Andrew F. Smith, 301–3 (Oxford and New York: Oxford University Press, 2004).

6. Deborah Valenze, "The Culture History of Food," in *Routledge International Handbook of Food Studies*, ed. Ken Albala, 101–13 (London and New York: Routledge, 2013). Histories of foods, as Valenze points out, drew much of their inspiration early on from anthropological studies, and the two fields remain close. See Robert T. Dirks and Gina Hunter, "The Anthropology of Food," in *Routledge International Handbook of Food Studies*, ed. Ken Albala, 3–13 (London and New York: Routledge, 2013).

7. John Gregory Bourke, "The Folk Foods of the Rio Grande Valley and of Northern Mexico," *Journal of American Folklore* 8 (1895): 41–71. Brillat-Savarin

wove together art and science and Epicurean philosophy and remains much admired to this day. See Jean Anthelme Brillat-Savarin, *The Physiology of Taste, or Meditations on Transcendental Gastronomy*, trans. Arthur Machen (New York: Dover, 1960).

8. Arthur Goss, *Dietary Studies in New Mexico in 1895*, U.S. Department of Agriculture Office of Experiment Stations Bulletin 40 (Washington, DC: U.S. Government Printing Office, 1897); Goss, *Nutrition Investigations in New Mexico in 1897*, U.S. Department of Agriculture Office of Experiment Stations Bulletin 54 (Washington, DC: U.S. Government Printing Office, 1898).

9. "Intelligence gathering" might be a more apt label for Bourke's ethnographic studies. His regiment, the Third Cavalry, fought Indians throughout his thirteen years of service with it.

10. John Gregory Bourke, "The Urine Dance of the Zuni Indians of New Mexico," in *Annual Meeting of the American Association for the Advancement of Science* (Ann Arbor, MI: Privately printed and distributed with the author's compliments, 1885); Bourke, *Compilation of Notes and Memoranda Bearing upon the Use of Human Ordure and Human Urine* (N.p.: Privately printed, 1888).

11. Bourke, "Folk Foods of the Rio Grande Valley," 67–68.

12. A saturated fat has no double bonds between the carbon atoms of the fatty-acid chain and is thereby fully saturated with hydrogen atoms. Such fats tend to be solid at room temperature. A diet rich in saturated fats increases the risks of atherosclerosis (hardening of the arteries) and coronary heart disease.

13. *Queso de tuna*, or prickly pear cheese, consists of the fruit of the prickly pear boiled down to a syrupy paste.

14. H. B. Frissell, "Dietary Studies among the Negroes in 1897," in *Dietary Studies of Negroes in Eastern Virginia in 1897 and 1898*, by H. B. Frissell and Isabel Bevier, U.S. Department of Agriculture Office of Experiment Stations Bulletin 71 (Washington, DC: U.S. Government Printing Office, 1899).

15. E. Richards and A. Shapleigh, "Dietary Studies in Philadelphia and Chicago, 1892–93," in *Dietary Studies in Boston and Springfield, Mass., Philadelphia, Pa., and Chicago, Ill.*, ed. Lydia Southard and R. D. Milner, U.S. Department of Agriculture Office of Experiment Stations Bulletin 129 (Washington, DC: U.S. Government Printing Office, 1903).

16. W. O. Atwater and A. P. Bryant, *Dietary Studies in Chicago in 1895 and 1896*, U.S. Department of Agriculture Office of Experiment Stations Bulletin 55 (Washington, DC: U.S. Government Printing Office, 1898).

17. Charles E. Wait, "Dietary Studies of Families Living in the Mountain Region of Eastern Tennessee," in *Dietary Studies in Rural Regions in Vermont, Tennessee, and Georgia*, by J. L. Hills, Charles E. Wait, and H. C. White, U.S. Department of Agriculture Office of Experiment Stations Bulletin 221 (Washington, DC: U.S. Department of Agriculture, Office of Experiment Stations, 1909), 24.
  The area known as the Chilhowee Mountains encompasses ridges jutting in a generally northwesterly direction from the Great Smoky Range of the East Tennessee–North Carolina border.

18. Carpenter, "Life and Times of W. O. Atwater," 1710S–11S; see also, for example, Isabel Bevier, *Nutrition Investigations in Pittsburgh, Pa., 1894–1896*, U.S. Department of Agriculture Office of Experiment Stations Bulletin 52 (Washington, DC: U.S. Government Printing Office, 1898), 30–31.

19. Richards and Shapleigh, "Dietary Studies in Philadelphia and Chicago."

20. Atwater and Bryant, *Dietary Studies in Chicago in 1895 and 1896*; W. O. Atwater and C. D. Woods, *Dietary Studies in New York City in 1896 and 1897*, U.S. Department of Agriculture Office of Experiment Stations Bulletin 116 (Washington, DC: U.S. Department of Agriculture, Office of Experiment Stations, 1902); W. O. Atwater and C. D. Woods, *Dietary Studies in New York City in 1895 and 1896*, U.S. Department of Agriculture Office of Experiment Stations Bulletin 46 (Washington, DC: U.S. Government Printing Office, 1898); Bevier, *Nutrition Investigations in Pittsburgh*.

21. W. O. Atwater and C. D. Woods, *Dietary Studies with Reference to the Food of the Negro in Alabama in 1895 and 1896*, U.S. Department of Agriculture Office of Experiment Stations Bulletin 38 (Washington, DC: U.S. Department of Agriculture, Office of Experiment Stations, 1897); H. B. Frissell and Isabel Bevier, *Dietary Studies of Negroes in Eastern Virginia in 1897 and 1898*, U.S. Department of Agriculture Office of Experiment Stations Bulletin 71 (Washington, DC: U.S. Government Printing Office, 1899).

22. Atwater and Woods, *Dietary Studies with Reference to the Food of the Negro*.

23. Atwater and Woods, *Dietary Studies in New York City in 1896 and 1897*; Atwater and Woods, *Dietary Studies in New York City in 1895 and 1896*.

24. Betty B. Peterkin, "Food Consumption Research: Parade of Survey Greats," *Journal of Nutrition* 124, no. S9 (September 1994): 1836S–42S.

25. Of course, none of these calculations would have been necessary had researchers measured individual food consumption directly. The idea was certainly not a foreign one. Early studies included individual dietaries, but the stumbling block was the expense. Simply put, the cost of monitoring what every member of the family personally ate was far greater than the cost of weighing the household's groceries. Modern nutritionists get around this issue and study individuals' food consumption thanks to such instruments as recall questionnaires and food diaries. These devices trim research costs by making subjects responsible for reporting their own food intakes. Unfortunately, subjects usually do not report everything that they eat.

26. Prior to 1917, the nutritional value of minerals went unreported, and vitamins awaited discovery.

27. A. M. Mayer, "Historical Changes in the Mineral Content of Fruits and Vegetables," *British Food Journal* 99 (1997): 207–11.

28. J. M. Hodgson, B. H. Hsu-Hage, and M. L. Wahlqvist, "Food Variety as a Quantitative Descriptor of Food Intake," *Ecology of Food and Nutrition* 32 (1994): 137.

29. H. B. Gibson, S. Calvert, and D. W. May, *Dietary Studies at the University of Missouri in 1895*, Office of Experiment Stations Bulletin 31 (Washington, DC: U.S. Government Printing Office, 1896); J. L. Hills, Charles E. Wait, and H. C. White, *Dietary Studies in Rural Regions in Vermont, Tennessee, and Georgia*, U.S. Department of Agriculture Office of Experiment Stations Bulletin 221 (Washington, DC: U.S. Government Printing Office, 1909).

30. Winthrop E. Stone, *Dietary Studies at Purdue University, Lafayette, Ind., in 1895*, U.S. Department of Agriculture Office of Experiment Stations Bulletin 32 (Washington, DC: U.S. Department of Agriculture, Office of Experiment Stations, 1896).

31. Robert T. Dirks and Nancy Duran, "African American Dietary Patterns at the Beginning of the 20th Century," *Journal of Nutrition* 131 (2001): 1881–89.

32. John W. Bennett, Harvey L. Smith, and Herbert Passin, "Food and Culture in Southern Illinois—a Preliminary Report," *American Sociological Review* 7 (1942): 645–60.

33. The threshold is arbitrary, but it usually produces a short list of exceptionally popular items.

CHAPTER 2: MOUNTAINEERS AND A NUTRITION TRANSITION IN APPALACHIA

1. S. F. Du, B. Lu, F. Zhai, and B. M. Popkin, "A New Stage of the Nutrition Transition in China," *Public Health Nutrition* 5 (2002): 169–74; B. M. Popkin and S. Du, "Dynamics of the Nutrition Transition toward the Animal Foods Sector in China and Its Implications: A Worried Perspective," *Journal of Nutrition* 133 (2003): 389S–906S.

2. Adam Drewnowski and Barry M. Popkin, "The Nutrition Transition: New Trends in the Global Diet," *Nutrition Reviews* 55, no. 2 (1997): 31–43; B. M. Popkin, "The Nutrition Transition in Low-Income Countries: An Emerging Crisis," *Nutrition Reviews* 52 (1994): 285–98.

3. Charles E. Wait, *Dietary Studies at the University of Tennessee in 1895*, U.S. Department of Agriculture Office of Experiment Stations Bulletin 29 (Washington, DC: U.S. Government Printing Office, 1896); Wait, *Nutritional Investigations at the University of Tennessee in 1896 and 1897*, U.S. Department of Agriculture Office of Experiment Stations Bulletin 53 (Washington, DC: U.S. Government Printing Office, 1898).

4. Charles E. Wait, "Dietary Studies of Families Living in the Mountain Region of Eastern Tennessee," in *Dietary Studies in Rural Regions in Vermont, Tennessee, and Georgia*, by J. L. Hills, Charles E. Wait, and H. C. White, U.S. Department of Agriculture Office of Experiment Stations Bulletin 221 (Washington, DC: U.S. Government Printing Office, 1909), 21–116.
   Horace Kephart characterized the Mountaineers of East Tennessee ethnographically as a distinct people. They did not refer to themselves, however, as "Mountaineers." They called themselves "Mountain People." Horace Kephart, *Our Southern Highlanders: A Narrative of Adventure in the Southern Appalachians and a Study of Life among the Mountaineers* (Knoxville: University of Tennessee Press, 1913), 280.

5. H. C. White, "Dietary Studies in Georgia," in *Dietary Studies in Rural Regions in Vermont, Tennessee, and Georgia*, by J. L. Hills, Charles E. Wait, and H. C. White, U.S. Department of Agriculture Office of Experiment Stations Bulletin 221 (Washington, DC: U.S. Government Printing Office, 1909), 117–36.

6. Wait, "Dietary Studies of Families Living in the Mountain Region," 22.

7. Ibid., 83.

8. Emily Stevens Maclachlan, "The Diet Pattern of the South: A Study in Rural Sociology" (master's thesis, University of North Carolina, 1932), 14–22.

9. Sam Bowers Hilliard, *Hog Meat and Hoecake: Food Supply in the Old South, 1840–1860* (Carbondale: Southern Illinois University Press, 1972), 38–40.

10. Maclachlan, "Diet Pattern of the South," 20.

11. Maclachlan, "Diet Pattern of the South," 20; Joe G. Taylor, *Eating, Drinking, and Visiting in the South* (Baton Rouge: Louisiana State University Press, 1982), 11.

12. Eliot Wigginton, ed., *The Foxfire Book: Hog Dressing; Log Cabin Building; Mountain Crafts and Foods; Planting by the Signs; Snake Lore, Hunting Tales, Faith Healing; Moonshining; and Other Affairs of Plain Living* (Garden City, NY: Doubleday, 1972), 161.

13. Treatment with lime or ash also initiates a process called nixtamalization. It renders corn easier to grind, amplifies its flavor and aroma, and increases its nutritional value by freeing otherwise-bound niacin for absorption by the body. See Allan Davidson, *The Oxford Companion to Food* (Oxford: Oxford University Press, 1999), 534.

14. Taylor, *Eating, Drinking, and Visiting*, 10.

15. Linda Garland Page and Eliot Wigginton, eds., *The Foxfire Book of Appalachian Cookery* (New York: Gramercy Books, 1984), 185.

16. Taylor, *Eating, Drinking, and Visiting*, 22.

17. Maclachlan, "Diet Pattern of the South," 107.

18. Ibid.

19. Horace Kephart, *Our Southern Highlanders: A Narrative of Adventure in the Southern Appalachians and a Study of Life among the Mountaineers* (Knoxville: University of Tennessee Press, 1913).

20. White, "Dietary Studies in Georgia."

21. Creighton Lee Calhoun, *Old Southern Apples* (Blacksburg, VA: McDonald and Woodward, 1995), 256.

22. See Wait, "Dietary Studies of Families Living in the Mountain Region," 82–104.

23. See chapter 6 for examples of caloric consumption by men employed as lumberjacks.

24. White, "Dietary Studies in Georgia," 136.

25. Wait, "Dietary Studies of Families Living in the Mountain Region," 114.

26. Ibid.

27. See ibid., 35–82.

28. Ibid., 113.

29. Wait, *Dietary Studies at the University of Tennessee*, 25–28; Wait, *Nutritional Investigations at the University of Tennessee*, 15–18; White, "Dietary Studies in Georgia," 123–24.

30. White, "Dietary Studies in Georgia," 123.

31. Wait, *Dietary Studies at the University of Tennessee*; Wait, *Nutritional Investigations at the University of Tennessee*; White, "Dietary Studies in Georgia."

32. Drewnowski and Popkin, "Nutrition Transition"; Popkin, "Nutrition Transition in Low-Income Countries"; Popkin, "The Nutrition Transition and Obesity in the Developing World," *Journal of Nutrition* 131 (2001): 871S–73S; Popkin, "The Nutrition Transition: An Overview of World Patterns of Change," *Nutrition Reviews* 62 (2004): S140–S43.

33. Urban working-class households consumed 425 g/m/d, but if potatoes are discounted, their vegetable use amounted to slightly less than Maryville's.

34. Wait, "Dietary Studies of Families Living in the Mountain Region," 111.

35. Sidney Andrews, *The South since the War: As Shown by Fourteen Weeks of Travel and Observation in Georgia and the Carolinas* (Boston: Tickner and Fields, 1866), 181–82.

CHAPTER 3: AFRICAN AMERICANS AND SOUL FOODS

1. See Cathryn Boyd Burke and Susan P. Raia, *Soul and Traditional Southern Food Practices, Customs, and Holidays*, Ethnic and Regional Food Practices (Chicago: American Dietetic Association; Alexandria, VA: American Diabetes Association, 1995).

2. Ibid., 8.

3. W. O. Atwater and C. D. Woods, *Dietary Studies with Reference to the Food of the Negro in Alabama in 1895 and 1896*, U.S. Department of Agriculture Office of Experiment Stations Bulletin 38 (Washington, DC: U.S. Department of Agriculture, Office of Experiment Stations, 1897); Isabel Bevier, "Dietary Studies among the

Negroes in 1898," in *Dietary Studies of Negroes in Eastern Virginia in 1897 and 1898*, by H. B. Frissell and Isabel Bevier, U.S. Department of Agriculture Office of Experiment Stations Bulletin 71 (Washington, DC: U.S. Government Printing Office, 1899); H. B. Frissell, "Dietary Studies among the Negroes in 1897," in *Dietary Studies of Negroes in Eastern Virginia in 1897 and 1898*, by H. B. Frissell and Isabel Bevier, U.S. Department of Agriculture Office of Experiment Stations Bulletin 71 (Washington, DC: U.S. Government Printing Office, 1899).

4. Atwater and his colleagues seldom saw beef on the hotel menu when they visited Tuskegee. See Atwater and Woods, *Dietary Studies with Reference to the Food of the Negro*, 20.

5. Frissell, "Dietary Studies among the Negroes in 1897."

6. Bevier, "Dietary Studies among the Negroes in 1898." Elizabeth City County no longer exits. It merged with the city of Hampton in 1952.

7. Frissell, "Dietary Studies among the Negroes in 1897," 7.

8. Bevier, who would go on to become the founder of the Department of Household Science at the University of Illinois, studied with Ellen Richards at the Massachusetts Institute of Technology. See Juliet Lita Bane, *The Story of Isabel Bevier* (Peoria, IL: C. A. Bennett, 1955).

9. Ellen H. Richards and Amelia Shapleigh, "Dietary Studies in Philadelphia and Chicago, 1892–93," in *Dietary Studies in Boston and Springfield, Mass., Philadelphia, Pa., and Chicago, Ill.*, ed. Lydia Southard and R. D. Milner, U.S. Department of Agriculture Office of Experiment Stations Bulletin 129 (Washington, DC: U.S. Government Printing Office, 1903), 37–98.

10. S. E. Forman, *Conditions of Living among the Poor*, Bulletin of the Bureau of Labor 64 (Washington, DC: U.S. Government Printing Office, 1906).

11. Alfred F. Hess and Lester J. Unger, "The Diet of the Negro Mother in New York City," *Journal of the American Medical Association* 70, no. 13 (1918): 900–902.

12. R. T. Steinbock, "Rickets and Osteomalacia," in *The Cambridge World History of Human Disease*, ed. Kenneth F. Kiple (Cambridge: Cambridge University Press, 1993): 978–80.

13. Institute for Colored Youth at Cheyney, *Applied Domestic Science Daily Menus for the School Year and a Dietary Study for October* (Philadelphia: Press of E. A. Wright, 1909).

14. Ibid.

15. Fannie Merritt Farmer, *Boston Cooking-School Cook Book* (Boston: Little, Brown, 1896).

16. Sweet potatoes appear in approximately 40 percent of the food inventories taken in the homes of southern whites.

17. Joint FAO/WHO/UNU Expert Consultation, *Energy and Protein Requirements*, World Health Organization Technical Report Series 724 (Geneva: World Health Organization, 1985), sec. 6.1.

18. Booker T. Washington, *Up from Slavery: An Autobiography* (New York: Doubleday, 1901), 115.

19. Ibid.

20. Ibid.

21. Tracy N. Poe, "The Origins of Soul Food in Black Urban Identity: Chicago, 1915–1947," *Amercan Studies International* 37, no. 1 (1999): 4–33.

CHAPTER 4: RICH AND POOR AND THE SEASONALITY OF DIET

1. Harvey A. Levenstein, *Revolution at the Table: The Transformation of the American Diet* (New York: Oxford University Press, 1988).

2. See ibid., 23.

3. "Hungry months" and similar labels such as "hunger season" refer to annual periods of semi-starvation or undernutrition, usually accompanied by a small and sometimes nearly imperceptible increase in death rates. Seasonal hungers have been common to parts of African and other areas of the Third World in the recent past but are less so today. Generally, the concept of seasonal hunger has not been applied to seasonal deficiencies in the United States.

4. Levenstein, *Revolution at the Table*, 12–13.

5. Ibid., 14.

6. W. O. Atwater and A. P. Bryant, *Dietary Studies in Chicago in 1895 and 1896*, U.S. Department of Agriculture Office of Experiment Stations Bulletin 55 (Washington, DC: U.S. Government Printing Office, 1898), 66–69.

7. In addition to the three inventories collected in the Chicago area, OES fieldworkers documented middle-class eating habits among the families of

professional chemists (see W. O. Atwater, *Methods and Results of Investigations on the Chemistry and Economy of Food*, U.S. Department of Agriculture Office of Experiment Stations Bulletin 21 [Washington, DC: U.S. Government Printing Office, 1895]; W. O. Atwater and C. D. Woods, "Studies of Dietaries," in *Connecticut Storrs Station Report for 1894* [Storrs, CT: Storrs Agricultural Experiment Station, 1894], 174–204; Atwater and Woods, "Food Investigations and Publications," in *Storrs Agricultural Experiment Station Bulletin* 15 [1895], 3–15; C. D. Woods, "A Study of Dietaries," in *Connecticut Storrs Station Report* [Storrs, CT: Storrs Agricultural Experiment Station, 1891], 90–106), college professors (Winthrop E. Stone, *Dietary Studies at Purdue University, Lafayette, Ind., in 1895*, U.S. Department of Agriculture Office of Experiment Stations Bulletin 32 [Washington, DC: U.S. Department of Agriculture, Office of Experiment Stations, 1896]; H. S. Grindley and J. I. Sammis, "Dietary Studies at the University of Illinois," in *Nutritional Investigations at the University of Illinois, North Dakota Agricultural College, and Lake Erie College, Ohio, 1896 to 1900*, by H. S. Grindley, J. L. Sammis, E. F. Ladd, Isabel Bevier, and E. C. Sprague, U.S. Department of Agriculture Office of Experiment Stations Bulletin 91 [Washington, DC: U.S. Government Printing Office, 1900], 7–20; J. L. Hills, "Dietary Studies in Vermont Farmers' Families," in *Dietary Studies in Rural Regions in Vermont, Tennessee, and Georgia*, by J. L. Hills, Charles E. Wait, and H. C. White, U.S. Department of Agriculture Office of Experiment Stations Bulletin 221 [Washington, DC: U.S. Department of Agriculture, Office of Experiment Stations, 1909], 11–13), a New York City social worker (W. O. Atwater and C. D. Woods, *Dietary Studies in New York City in 1895 and 1896*, U.S. Department of Agriculture Office of Experiment Stations Bulletin 46 [Washington, DC: U.S. Government Printing Office, 1898], 62), and a Pittsburgh lawyer (Isabel Bevier, *Nutrition Investigations in Pittsburgh, Pa., 1894–1896*, U.S. Department of Agriculture Office of Experiment Stations Bulletin 52 [Washington, DC: U.S. Government Printing Office, 1898], 12–17).

8. Stone, *Dietary Studies at Purdue University*, 12–15; Atwater and Woods, *Dietary Studies in New York City in 1895 and 1896*, 113–15; Bevier, *Nutrition Investigations in Pittsburgh*, 12–15; Grindley and Sammis, "Dietary Studies at the University of Illinois," 15–16.

9. Donna R. Gabaccia, *We Are What We Eat: Ethnic Food and the Making of Americans* (Cambridge, MA: Harvard University Press, 1998), 125.

10. Ibid., 126–27; Levenstein, *Revolution at the Table*, 56–57.

11. A composed salad consisted of fresh or canned vegetables and fruits with nuts and perhaps some cottage cheese, all artfully arranged on small, decorative plates.

12. Richard J. Hooker, *Food and Drink in America: A History* (Indianapolis, IN: Bobbs-Merrill, 1981), 238–39; Levenstein, *Revolution at the Table*, 5.

13. Hooker, *Food and Drink in America*, 241.

14. Ibid., 222.

15. Ibid., 229.

16. Ibid., 232–33.

17. Ibid., 126.

18. Ellen H. Richards and Marion Talbot, *Food as a Factor in Student Life* (Chicago: University of Chicago Press, 1894).

19. Ibid., 16–22.

20. Likely refers to Schumacher's Parched Farinose, a packaged product touted on an undated advertising card as "the Perfect Type of Food—Rich in Gluten, Cerm [*sic*], Gum and Sugar. Cooks in 2 Minutes—Unsurpassed as a Breakfast Dish."

21. A steamed dish of sponge cake and raisins covered with a mixture of eggs and milk.

22. Richards and Talbot, *Food as a Factor*.

23. The middle-class household dietaries yielded slightly higher values primarily because the researchers made no allowance for waste.

24. Levenstein, *Revolution at the Table*, 23.

25. Ellen H. Richards and Amelia Shapleigh, "Dietary Studies in Philadelphia and Chicago, 1892–93," in *Dietary Studies in Boston and Springfield, Mass., Philadelphia, Pa., and Chicago, Ill.*, ed. Lydia Southard and R. D. Milner, U.S. Department of Agriculture Office of Experiment Stations Bulletin 129 (Washington, DC: U.S. Government Printing Office, 1903), 37–98.

26. Atwater and Woods, *Dietary Studies in New York City in 1895 and 1896*; Atwater and Bryant, *Dietary Studies in Chicago in 1895 and 1896*; W. O. Atwater and C. D. Woods, *Dietary Studies in New York City in 1896 and 1897*, U.S. Department of Agriculture Office of Experiment Stations Bulletin 116 (Washington, DC: U.S. Department of Agriculture, Office of Experiment Stations, 1902).

27. S. E. Forman, *Conditions of Living among the Poor*, Bulletin of the Bureau of Labor 64 (Washington, DC: U.S. Government Printing Office, 1906).

28. Richards and Shapleigh, "Dietary Studies in Philadelphia and Chicago," 37–40, 64. Settlement houses, such as Hull House, were established in impoverished urban neighborhoods throughout the United States. The houses originated in the 1880s in connection with a social movement intended to aid society's poor through exposure to practical and mentally stimulating aspects of American culture. Settlement houses were populated with settlement workers, mostly well-educated women dedicated to improving the lives of the neighborhood's poor.

29. Ibid., 40–44.

30. K. Stitt, "Nutritive Value of Diets Today and Fifty Years Ago," *Journal of the American Dietetic Association* 36 (1960): 433–40. Butter, lard, and salt pork were the most frequently used fats. According to Stitt, an estimated 82 percent of all households used butter. Seventy-six percent used lard. Salt pork was included in the diets of approximately 42 percent. Suet was used by around 10 percent of households.

31. Forman, *Conditions of Living among the Poor*.

32. Ibid., 593–94.

33. Ibid., 603.

34. Ibid., 603–4.

35. Ibid., 605.

36. Atwater and Woods, *Dietary Studies in New York City in 1895 and 1896*; Atwater and Woods, *Dietary Studies in New York City in 1896 and 1897*.

37. Atwater and Woods, *Dietary Studies in New York City in 1896 and 1897*; see Atwater and Woods, *Dietary Studies in New York City in 1895 and 1896*.

38. Not counting immigrants, the collection includes five dietaries collected during the fall, three during the winter, thirteen during the spring, and six during the summer.

39. Caroline Goodyear, "Household Budgets of the Poor: An Inquiry into the Dietary Standards and Habits of a Group of Tenement House Families in New York City," *Charities and the Commons* 16, no. 4 (1906): 191–97.

40. C. F. Langworthy, "Food and Diet in the United States," in *Yearbook of the United States Department of Agriculture* (1908): 361–78.

41. Hooker, *Food and Drink in America*, 218.

42. Levenstein, *Revolution at the Table*, 26–29.

43. Elizabeth W. Etheridge, "Pellagra," in *The Cambridge World History of Human Disease*, ed. Kenneth F. Kiple (Cambridge: Cambridge University Press, 1993).

44. Dorothy Dickins, *A Nutrition Investigation of Negro Tenants in the Yazoo Mississippi Delta*, in Mississippi Agricultural Experiment Station Bulletin 254 (Agricultural College: Mississippi Agricultural Experiment Station, 1928).

45. W. O. Atwater and C. D. Woods, *Dietary Studies with Reference to the Food of the Negro in Alabama in 1895 and 1896*, U.S. Department of Agriculture Office of Experiment Stations Bulletin 38 (Washington, DC: U.S. Department of Agriculture, Office of Experiment Stations, 1897), 19.

46. Booker T. Washington, *Up from Slavery: An Autobiography* (New York: Doubleday, 1901), 66.

47. Dickins, *Nutrition Investigation of Negro Tenants*, 11.

48. Atwater and Woods, *Dietary Studies with Reference to the Food of the Negro*.

49. Ibid., 68.

50. The WHO standard is 0.75 g/kg/m/d. This translates to 51 g/m/d. The current U.S. standard is 0.66 g/m/d per kilogram of body weight. See N. S. Scrimshaw, "Human Protein Requirements: A Brief Update," in *Food and Nutrition Bulletin* 17, no. 3 (September 1996): 185–90; Institute of Medicine and National Academy of Sciences, *Dietary Reference Intakes for Energy, Carbohydrate, Fiber, Fat, Fatty Acids, Cholesterol, Protein, and Amino Acids: A Report of the Panel on Macronutrients, Subcommittees on Upper Reference Levels of Nutrients and Interpretation and Uses of Dietary Reference Intakes and the Standing Committee on the Scientific Evaluation of Dietary Reference Intakes* (Washington, DC: National Academies Press, 2002).

The WHO standard seems preferable here because it was developed with economically undeveloped regions in mind. With respect to work and disease patterns, American environments at the beginning of the twentieth century were more like those of underdeveloped countries than those of the contemporary United States.

51. Charles E. Wait, "Dietary Studies of Families Living in the Mountain Region of Eastern Tennessee," in *Dietary Studies in Rural Regions in Vermont, Tennessee, and Georgia*, by J. L. Hills, Charles E. Wait, and H. C. White, U.S. Department of Agriculture Office of Experiment Stations Bulletin 221 (Washington, DC: U.S. Government Printing Office, 1909), 21–116.

52. J. A. Albright, "Pellagra in Tennessee," in *Pellagra*, ed. K. J. Carpenter (Stroudsburg, PA: Hutchinson Ross, 1981).

53. See Etheridge, "Pellagra."

54. J. Goldberger, G. A. Wheeler, E. Sydenstricker, and W. I. King, *A Study of Endemic Pellagra in Some Cotton-Mill Villages of South Carolina*, U.S. Public Health Service, Hygienic Laboratory Bulletin 153 (Washington, DC: U.S. Government Printing Office, 1929).

55. K. J. Carpenter, "Editors Comments on Papers 31 through 37," in *Pellagra*, ed. K. J. Carpenter (Stroudsburg, PA: Hutchinson Ross, 1981), 272.

56. The nixtamalization of corn to make hominy prevents pellagra (see chapter 2). However, food inventories indicate that by the end of the nineteenth century, only about 10 percent of American households were consuming hominy or other nixtamalized corn products. Hominy consumption in east Tennessee appears to have been under 10 percent. There is no telling whether more or less hominy was consumed at an earlier date.

57. Based on a total of twenty-seven dietaries—five fall, five winter, six spring, and eleven summer. See Atwater and Woods, *Dietary Studies in New York City in 1895 and 1896*; Atwater and Woods, *Dietary Studies in New York City in 1896 and 1897*.

58. The term *trucker* at the time referred to a person who pushed a hand truck.

59. Richard Osborn Cummings, *The American and His Food: A History of Food Habits in the United States* (Chicago: University of Chicago Press, 1940), 75–76.

60. Richard H. Steckel, "Slave Height Profiles from Coastwise Manifests," *Explorations in Economic History* 16 (1979): 363–80. Other early, influential works in the field of anthropometric history include Roderick Floud, Kenneth Wachter, and Annabel Gregory, *Height, Health, and History: Nutritional Status in the United Kingdom, 1750–1980* (Cambridge: Cambridge University Press, 1990); Robert W. Fogel, Stanley L. Engerman, and James Trussell, "Exploring the Uses of Data on Height," *Social Science History* 6, no. 4 (1982): 401–21; John Komlos, *Nutrition and Economic Development in the Eighteenth-Century Habsburg Monarchy: An Anthropometric History* (Princeton, NJ: Princeton University Press, 1989).

61. Average adult stature is such a good measure of prior nutritional and disease experiences that it can be used to retrodict average levels of childhood mortality. This is of particular significance for the Gilded Age, toward the end of which at least half of all childhood deaths occurred on account of nutritionally sensitive diseases such as measles, diarrheas, tuberculosis, and whooping cough. Michael R. Haines and Richard H. Steckel, *Childhood Mortality and Nutritional Status as Indicators of*

Standard of Living: Evidence from World War I Recruits in the United States, National Bureau of Economic Research Working Paper Series on Historical Factors in Long-Run Growth, Historical Paper 121 (Cambridge, MA: National Bureau of Economic Research, 2000), 9.

62. Richard H. Steckel, "Heights and Health in the United States, 1710–1950," in *Stature, Living Standards, and Economic Development*, ed. John Komlos (Chicago: University of Chicago Press, 1994), 153–70.

63. The precise difference was 2.2 cm (0.88 inches). Middle-class inductees from professional backgrounds measured in at an average 175.5 cm (5 ft 10 in). Guardsmen from the ranks of the unskilled measured an average 173.3 cm (5 ft 8 in). The average height of clerical and skilled workers fell in between the two at 174 cm (5 ft 9 in). These findings pertained specifically to the Ohio National Guard. However, the researchers found no reason to believe these differences were peculiar to Ohio. Richard H. Steckel and Donald R. Haurin, "Health and Nutrition in the American Midwest: Evidence from the Height of Ohio National Guardsmen, 1850–1910," in *Stature, Living Standards, and Economic Development*, ed. John Komlos (Chicago: University of Chicago Press, 1994), 117–28.

64. Levenstein, *Revolution at the Table*, 25.

65. Richard Longhurst and Philip Payne, "Seasonal Aspects of Nutrition," in *Seasonal Dimensions to Rural Poverty*, ed. Robert Chambers, Richard Longhurst, and Arnold Pacey (Totowa, NJ: Allanheld, Osmun, 1981), 45–51; Ellen Messer, "Season Hunger and Coping Strategies: An Anthropological Discussion," in *Coping with Seasonal Constraints*, ed. Rebecca Huss-Ashmore, John James Curry, and Robert K. Hitchcock (Philadelphia: MASCA, University Museum, University of Pennsylvania, 1989), 131–41.

CHAPTER 5: IMMIGRANTS' DIETS

1. Donna R. Gabaccia, *We Are What We Eat: Ethnic Food and the Making of Americans* (Cambridge, MA: Harvard University Press, 1998).

2. Ibid., 62.

3. The nationalities represented are Austrian, Bohemian, English, German, Hungarian, Irish, Italian, Polish, Romanian, Russian, Scots, Swedish, and Swiss.

4. The literature contains a total of twenty-nine German dietary and household budget studies.

5. Twenty-six studies documented Bohemian American eating habits. Five studies detailed food consumption among British Americans, twenty-four studies among Irish Americans, nine studies among Italian Americans, and nineteen studies among Russian Jewish Americans.

6. *Worldmark Encyclopedia of Cultures and Daily Life*, vol. 2, *Americas*, ed. Timothy L. Gall and Jeneen Hobby (Detroit, MI: Gale, 2009), s.v. "Italian Americans."

7. Ellen H. Richards and Amelia Shapleigh, "Dietary Studies in Philadelphia and Chicago, 1892–93," in *Dietary Studies in Boston and Springfield, Mass., Philadelphia, Pa., and Chicago, Ill.*, ed. Lydia Southard and R. D. Milner, U.S. Department of Agriculture Office of Experiment Stations Bulletin 129 (Washington, DC: U.S. Government Printing Office, 1903), 44–45.

8. Robert Coit Chapin, *The Standard of Living among Workingmen's Families in New York City* (New York: Charities Publication Committee, 1909; repr. New York: Arno Press, 1971), 159–60.

9. W. O. Atwater and A. P. Bryant, *Dietary Studies in Chicago in 1895 and 1896*, U.S. Department of Agriculture Office of Experiment Stations Bulletin 55 (Washington, DC: U.S. Government Printing Office, 1898); W. O. Atwater and C. D. Woods, *Dietary Studies in New York City in 1896 and 1897*, U.S. Department of Agriculture Office of Experiment Stations Bulletin 116 (Washington, DC: U.S. Department of Agriculture, Office of Experiment Stations, 1902).

10. Atwater and Woods, *Dietary Studies in New York City in 1896 and 1897*, 15.

11. Richards and Shapleigh, "Dietary Studies in Philadelphia and Chicago."

12. Chapin, *Standard of Living*, 137. This study included data from fifty-seven Italian American households.

13. Ibid., 139.

14. Ibid., 147. In contrast with budget studies, dietary studies did not systematically account for alcoholic beverages. Wine received only incidental mention. W. O. Atwater and his fellow chemists did not regard it as a proper food. Like many other middle-class Americans at the time, they condemned drinking wine and spirits as an unnecessary drain on household resources. Beer was another matter. Fieldworkers inventoried it, and among Italians they found it present in the kitchen almost as often as olive oil, tomatoes, and other commodities essential to Italian American cuisine. A comparison of immigrant dietaries showed that no one except Bohemians

drank beer at home more often than Italians. Note, however, that immigrants from Germany, Ireland, and several other European countries did not normally drink beer, wine, and spirits at home. Consequently, their drinking habits escaped the purview of investigators conducting household studies.

15. Atwater and Bryant, *Dietary Studies in Chicago in 1895 and 1896*, 15–16.

16. Atwater and Woods, *Dietary Studies in New York City in 1896 and 1897*, 40–42.

17. See Jane Ziegelman, *97 Orchard Street: An Edible History of Five Immigrant Families in One New York Tenement* (New York: Smithsonian Books/HarperCollins, 2010), 194.

18. Atwater and Bryant, *Dietary Studies in Chicago in 1895 and 1896*, 15–16.

19. Richard J. Hooker, *Food and Drink in America: A History* (Indianapolis, IN: Bobbs-Merrill, 1981), 291; Chapin, *Standard of Living*.

20. Veal, a primary food in the typical European American diet, did not show up often in food lists collected from Italian immigrants. This may have been an artifact of timing, seeing as the availability of veal at popular prices was limited to the spring calving season.

21. Missing from the list of foods in most European American homes were oatmeal, rye bread, and cakes.

22. Hasia R. Diner, *Hungering for America: Italian, Irish, and Jewish Foodways in the Age of Migration* (Cambridge, MA: Harvard University Press, 2001), 29.

23. W. O. Atwater, *Methods and Results of Investigations on the Chemistry and Economy of Food*, U.S. Department of Agriculture Office of Experiment Stations Bulletin 21 (Washington, DC: U.S. Government Printing Office, 1895), 1733.

24. Ibid.

25. Harvey A. Levenstein, "The American Response to Italian Food, 1880–1930," *Food and Foodways* 1, no. 1 (1985): 3.

26. Atwater, *Methods and Results*, 180.

27. "Russian American," *Wikipedia*, http://en.wikipedia.org/w/index.php?title=Russian_American&oldid=649943306.

28. Ibid.

29. *Shtetl* culture refers to the way of life in the small villages and towns that most Eastern European Jewish immigrants left behind. See Irving Cutler, "Jews," in *The Electronic Encyclopedia of Chicago*, ed. Janice L. Reiff, Ann Durkin Keating, and James R. Grossman (Chicago: Chicago Historical Society, 2005), http://www .encyclopedia.chicagohistory.org/pages/671.html.

30. Katarzyna Zechenterd, "Russians," in *The Electronic Encyclopedia of Chicago*, ed. Janice L. Reiff, Ann Durkin Keating, and James R. Grossman (Chicago: Chicago Historical Society, 2005), http://www.encyclopedia.chicagohistory.org/pages/1104 .html; Cutler, "Jews."

31. Atwater and Bryant, *Dietary Studies in Chicago in 1895 and 1896*, 10–11, 26–43.

32. Ibid.

33. Diner, *Hungering for America*, 163.

34. Average energy intake for immigrants represented in early dietaries came to 3,322 Cal/m/d.

35. Atwater and Bryant, *Dietary Studies in Chicago in 1895 and 1896*, 36.

36. Atwater and Bryant, *Dietary Studies in Chicago in 1895 and 1896*, 36; Chapin, *Standard of Living*, 156–57; Louise Moore, "The Food of Women Living Away from Their Families," in *The Food of Working Women in Boston*, ed. Lucile Eaves, Studies in Economic Relations of Women 10 (Boston: Wright and Potter, 1917), 96–97.

37. Atwater and Bryant, *Dietary Studies in Chicago in 1895 and 1896*, 38.

38. Atwater and Bryant, *Dietary Studies in Chicago in 1895 and 1896*, 36.

39. Chicago's mean (3,373 Cal/m/d) intake exceeded the average among Moscow-area peasants by a mere 100 Cal/m/d; see Atwater, *Methods and Results*, 178.

40. Ibid.

41. Chapin, *Standard of Living*, 138.

42. Hooker, *Food and Drink in America*, 287.

43. Atwater and Bryant, *Dietary Studies in Chicago in 1895 and 1896*, 43–65; Richards and Shapleigh, "Dietary Studies in Philadelphia and Chicago," 91.

44. Atwater and Bryant, *Dietary Studies in Chicago in 1895 and 1896*, 43.

45. Beer appeared under the heading "Food Accessories," an inappropriate label considering beer's centrality to the Bohemian table. See ibid., 43–65.

46. Ibid.

47. The table is based on data from a total of twenty-two households.

48. *Worldmark Encyclopedia of Cultures and Daily Life*, vol. 2, *Americas*, s.v. "Irish Americans."

49. Richards and Shapleigh, "Dietary Studies in Philadelphia and Chicago"; Atwater and Woods, *Dietary Studies in New York City in 1896 and 1897*; Isabel Bevier, *Nutrition Investigations in Pittsburgh, Pa., 1894–1896*, U.S. Department of Agriculture Office of Experiment Stations Bulletin 52 (Washington, DC: U.S. Government Printing Office, 1898).

50. Diner, *Hungering for America.*

51. Ibid., 132. Ziegelman (*97 Orchard Street*, 80–81), who also appears unaware of the OES dietaries, repeats Diner's story about the place of corned beef in the nineteenth-century Irish American kitchen.

52. Brian Murton, "Famine," in *The Cambridge World History of Food*, ed. Kenneth F. Kiple and Kriemhild Conee Ornelas (Cambridge: Cambridge University Press, 2000), 1412.

53. Allan Davidson, *The Oxford Companion to Food* (Oxford: Oxford University Press, 1999), 218.

54. Brid Mahon, *Land of Milk and Honey: The Story of Traditional Irish Food and Drink* (Cork, Ireland: Mercier Press, 1998), 127.

55. See Atwater and Bryant, *Dietary Studies in Chicago in 1895 and 1896*; Richards and Shapleigh, "Dietary Studies in Philadelphia and Chicago."

56. Calculated from German American dietaries contained in Atwater and Bryant, *Dietary Studies in Chicago in 1895 and 1896*; W. O. Atwater and C. D. Woods, *Dietary Studies in New York City in 1895 and 1896*, U.S. Department of Agriculture Office of Experiment Stations Bulletin 46 (Washington, DC: U.S. Government Printing Office, 1898); Richards and Shapleigh, "Dietary Studies in Philadelphia and Chicago."

57. Calculated from British and French Canadian dietaries contained in Atwater and Woods, *Dietary Studies in New York City in 1895 and 1896*; Bevier, *Nutrition*

Investigations in Pittsburgh; Richards and Shapleigh, "Dietary Studies in Philadelphia and Chicago."

58. Bridget Haggerty, "Celebrating St. Patrick's Day in Old Ireland," Irish Culture and Customs, http://www.irishcultureandcustoms.com/.

59. Compared to immigrant diets, those of second-generation families contained more energy (3,771 Cal/m/d versus 3,404 Cal/m/d), less animal protein (64 g/m/d versus 74 g/m/d), more total protein (125 g/m/d versus 117 g/m/d), less total fat (30 percent versus 36 percent), and less animal fat (26 percent versus 33 percent) relative to energy intake. See W. O. Atwater and A. P. Bryant, "Studies of Dietaries," in *Connecticut Storrs Station Report for 1896* (Storrs, CT: Storrs Agricultural Experiment Station, 1896), 117–58; Atwater and Woods, *Dietary Studies in New York City in 1895 and 1896*; Richards and Shapleigh, "Dietary Studies in Philadelphia and Chicago."

60. "British American," *Wikipedia*, http://en.wikipedia.org/w/index.php?title=British_American&oldid=649759185.

61. Both English and Scottish households are included. See Atwater and Woods, *Dietary Studies in New York City in 1895 and 1896*, 17–20, 51–55; Bevier, *Nutrition Investigations in Pittsburgh*, 22–31; Richards and Shapleigh, "Dietary Studies in Philadelphia and Chicago," 84–85.

62. Bevier, *Nutrition Investigations in Pittsburgh*, 22–31.

63. Diarmid Noël Paton, J. Craufurd Dunlop, and E. Inglis, *A Study of the Diet of the Labouring Classes in Edinburgh, Carried Out under the Auspices of the Town Council of the City of Edinburgh* (Edinburgh: Otto Schulze, 1902), 61.

64. Cf. W. O Atwater, "American and European Dietaries and Dietary Standards," in *Connecticut Storrs Station Report for 1891* (Storrs, CT: Storrs School Agricultural Experiment Station, 1891), 142. B. Seebohm Rowntree, *Poverty: A Study of Town Life* (New York: Howard Fertig, 1902), 97, 279.

65. Calculated from Paton, Dunlop, and Inglis, *Study of the Diet of the Labouring Classes*, 44–58.

66. Calculated from ibid.

67. Rowntree, *Poverty*, 279.

68. Calculated from Paton, Dunlop, and Inglis, *Study of the Diet of the Labouring Classes*, 44–58.

69. *Worldmark Encyclopedia of Cultures and Daily Life*, vol. 2, *Americas*, ed. Timothy L. Gall and Jeneen Hobby (Detroit, MI: Gale, 2009), s.v. "German Americans."

70. "German American," *Wikipedia*, http://en.wikipedia.org/w/index.php?title=German_American&oldid=650341691.

71. Ibid.

72. Richards and Shapleigh, "Dietary Studies in Philadelphia and Chicago."

73. Atwater and Woods, *Dietary Studies in New York City in 1896 and 1897*; Atwater and Woods, "Dietary Studies in New York City in 1895 and 1896."

74. Chapin, *Standard of Living*, 137.

75. Summarized in Atwater, *Methods and Results*, 163–73.

76. Ibid.

77. Ibid., 164.

78. Calculated from ibid., 176–79.

79. Werner Sombart, *Why Is There No Socialism in the United States?* (White Plains, NY: M. E. Sharpe, 1976).

80. Atwater, "American and European Dietaries," 143.

81. Ibid., 142.

82. See ibid.

83. See Atwater, *Methods and Results*, 178.

84. See ibid., 179.

85. See Atwater, "American and European Dietaries," 142.

86. See ibid., 143.

87. Richard H. Steckel and Donald R. Haurin, "Health and Nutrition in the American Midwest: Evidence from the Height of Ohio National Guardsmen, 1850–1910," in *Stature, Living Standards, and Economic Development*, ed. John Komlos (Chicago: University of Chicago Press, 1994), 153–70.

88. Richard H. Steckel, *Stature and Living Standards in the United States*, National Bureau of Economic Research Working Paper Series on Historical Factors in Long-Run Growth Working Paper 24 (Cambridge, MA: National Bureau of Economic Research, 1991), 29.

89. To turn things around, take French Canadians and Russian Jews. Both spent nearly the same amount of money, but the mean number of different items found in the market baskets of non-Orthodox Jews was considerably less than the number found in the French Canadians'.

90. Irish American families living in New York City spent no more on food in the second generation than in the first. As one would expect were variety strictly a matter of spending, members of both generations consumed about the same number of foods per week. These data, collected over ten-day stretches and thus omitted from the table, lend no support to the idea that acculturation or the process of Americanization worked independently toward broadening the range of foods in immigrant diets.

91. Obesity is usually defined these days with reference to body mass index (BMI).

92. M. S. Goel, E. P. McCarthy, R. S. Phillips, and C. C. Wee, "Obesity among US Immigrant Subgroups by Duration of Residence," *Journal of the American Medical Association* 292, no. 23 (2004): 2860–67.

CHAPTER 6: CONTRASTS

1. E. Mallinckrodt, *Dietary Studies with Harvard University Students*, U.S. Department of Agriculture Office of Experiment Stations Bulletin 152 (Washington, DC: U.S. Government Printing Office, 1905).

2. H. C. White, "Dietary Studies in Georgia," in *Dietary Studies in Rural Regions in Vermont, Tennessee, and Georgia*, by J. L. Hills, Charles E. Wait, and H. C. White, U.S. Department of Agriculture Office of Experiment Stations Bulletin 221 (Washington, DC: U.S. Government Printing Office, 1909), 121–23.

3. W. O. Atwater, *Methods and Results of Investigations on the Chemistry and Economy of Food*, U.S. Department of Agriculture Office of Experiment Stations Bulletin 21 (Washington, DC: U.S. Government Printing Office, 1895), 196–97.

4. Charles E. Wait, *Dietary Studies at the University of Tennessee in 1895*, U.S. Department of Agriculture Office of Experiment Stations Bulletin 29 (Washington, DC: U.S. Government Printing Office, 1896); Wait, *Nutritional Investigations at the University of Tennessee in 1896 and 1897*, U.S. Department of Agriculture Office of Experiment Stations Bulletin 53 (Washington, DC: U.S. Government Printing Office, 1898).

5. O. F. Tower, "Dietary Studies at Western Reserve University," *Western Reserve University Bulletin*, n.s., 4 (1901): 146–64; Ellen H. Richards and Marion Talbot, *Food*

as a Factor in Student Life (Chicago: University of Chicago Press, 1894); W. Jordan, *Dietary Studies at the Maine State College in 1895*, U.S. Department of Agriculture Office of Experiment Stations Bulletin 37 (Washington, DC: U.S. Department of Agriculture, Office of Experiment Stations, 1897); Isabel Bevier and E. C. Sprague, "Dietary Study at Lake Erie College, Painesville, Ohio," in *Nutritional Investigations at the University of Illinois, North Dakota Agricultural College, and Lake Erie College, Ohio, 1896 to 1900*, by H. S. Grindley, J. L. Sammis, E. F. Ladd, Isabel Bevier, and E. C. Sprague, U.S. Department of Agriculture Office of Experiment Stations Bulletin 91 (Washington, DC: U.S. Government Printing Office, 1900), 27–38.

6. Richards and Talbot, *Food as a Factor*, 7–9.

7. Tower, "Dietary Studies at Western Reserve University," 154.

8. Ibid., 146.

9. Dietaries for boarding clubs on campuses located in the Northeast are reported in H. B. Gibson, C. D. Woods, and W. O. Atwater, "Studies of Dietaries," in *Connecticut Storrs Station Report for 1893* (Storrs, CT: Storrs Agricultural Experiment Station, 1893), 185–87; W. O. Atwater and C. D. Woods, "Studies of Dietaries," in *Connecticut Storrs Station Report for 1894* (Storrs, CT: Storrs Agricultural Experiment Station, 1894), 183–94; W. O. Atwater and C. D. Woods, "Studies of Dietaries," in *Connecticut Storrs Station Report for 1895* (Storrs, CT: Storrs Agricultural Experiment Station, 1895), 166–70; Jordan, *Dietary Studies at the Maine State College*. For the midwestern schools, see Richards and Talbot, *Food as a Factor*; H. B. Gibson, S. Calvert, and D. W. May, *Dietary Studies at the University of Missouri in 1895*, U.S. Department of Agriculture Office of Experiment Stations Bulletin 31 (Washington, DC: U.S. Government Printing Office, 1896); E. F. Ladd, "Dietary Study of a Club of Women Students at North Dakota Agricultural College," in *Nutritional Investigations at the University of Illinois, North Dakota Agricultural College, and Lake Erie College, Ohio, 1896 to 1900*, by H. S. Grindley, J. L. Sammis, E. F. Ladd, Isabel Bevier, and E. C. Sprague, U.S. Department of Agriculture Office of Experiment Stations Bulletin 91 (Washington, DC: U.S. Government Print Office, 1900); Bevier and Sprague, "Dietary Study at Lake Erie College"; Tower, "Dietary Studies at Western Reserve University."

10. Dietaries for boarding clubs on southern campuses are reported in Wait, *Dietary Studies at the University of Tennessee*; Wait, *Nutritional Investigations at the University of Tennessee*; White, "Dietary Studies in Georgia."

11. Other items core to the typical diet on northern campuses but peripheral to the typical collegiate diet in the South included gelatin, chocolate, beets, squash, dried currants, and fruit preserves.

12. Other items core to the typical student diet in the North but missing from dietaries recorded in the South included cottolene, dairy cream, maple syrup, cocoa, carrots, parsnips, rhubarb, and spinach.

13. Of the seventy-eight foods recorded for colleges generally, eighteen with core status on one side of the Mason-Dixon Line were hardly ever served on the other. About 75 percent of the foods that students regularly used were common to both the North and the South.

14. The Missouri data shows that dairy consumption averaged just 36 g/m/d. See Gibson, Calvert, and May, *Dietary Studies at the University of Missouri.*

15. The consumption of beef fat by members of eating clubs at the Universities of Georgia and Tennessee averaged 15 g/m/d.

16. Atwater and Woods, "Studies of Dietaries" (1894); Gibson, Woods, and Atwater, "Studies of Dietaries"; Tower, "Dietary Studies at Western Reserve University."

17. Atwater and Woods, "Studies of Dietaries" (1894); Bevier and Sprague, "Dietary Study at Lake Erie College"; Gibson, Woods, and Atwater, "Studies of Dietaries."

18. The dietaries list thirty meat items served to males and twenty-one meat items offered to females.

19. Bevier and Sprague, "Dietary Study at Lake Erie College," 28.

20. W. O. Atwater, "American and European Dietaries and Dietary Standards," in *Connecticut Storrs Station Report for 1891* (Storrs, CT: Storrs School Agricultural Experiment Station, 1891), 150.

21. M. E. Jaffa, *Nutrition Investigations at the California Agricultural Experiment Station, 1896–1898,* U.S. Department of Agriculture Office of Experiment Stations Bulletin 84 (Washington, DC: U.S. Government Printing Office, 1900).

22. In retrospect, nutritionists have found this number improbably high. Very likely the "Golden Bears" were not the only ones helping themselves to the many dishes on offer at the players' training table. See P. B. Swan and K. J. Carpenter, "Myer E. Jaffa: Pioneering Chemist in the Food and Nutrition Sciences," *Bulletin for the History of Chemistry* 21 (1998): 51–57.

23. W. O. Atwater and A. P. Bryant, *Dietary Studies of University Boat Crews*, U.S. Department of Agriculture Office of Experiment Stations Bulletin 75 (Washington, DC: U.S. Government Printing Office, 1900).

24. Ibid., 60–63.

25. The varsity team, for example, consumed 321 g (11 oz.) of milk per man per day and practically as much cream.

26. The drink had almost no nutritional value. See Atwater and Bryant, *Dietary Studies of University Boat Crews*, 32.

27. The usual ration amounted to 330 g/m/d (11.6 oz./m/d). The University of California's football players drank porter, a darker and slightly stronger brew than most.

28. Ladd, "Dietary Study of a Club of Women."

29. There were exceptions, however. For example, at the University of Chicago and at Lake Erie College, researchers noted an occasional pork roast inserted into an otherwise beefy diet. See Richards and Talbot, *Food as a Factor*; Bevier and Sprague, "Dietary Study at Lake Erie College."

30. "Swift Refrigerator Line," *Wikipedia*, http://en.wikipedia.org/w/index.php?title=Swift_Refrigerator_Line&oldid=629527710.

31. Richard J. Hooker, *Food and Drink in America: A History* (Indianapolis, IN: Bobbs-Merrill, 1981), 21–22.

32. See Upton Sinclair, *The Jungle* (New York: Jungle Publishing Company, 1906).

33. Quoted in Harvey A. Levenstein, "The American Response to Italian Food, 1880–1930," *Food and Foodways* 1, no. 1 (1985): 7.

34. Richards and Talbot, *Food as a Factor*, 9.

35. Protein consumption averaged 63 g/m/d. See Bevier and Sprague, "Dietary Study at Lake Erie College," 33.

36. Protein consumption here averaged 56 g/m/d. See Ladd, "Dietary Study of a Club of Women Students," 25.

37. Tower, "Dietary Studies at Western Reserve University."

38. See Atwater and Woods, "Studies of Dietaries" (1894), 191–94; Gibson, Woods, and Atwater, "Studies of Dietaries," 185–87.

39. Richards and Talbot, *Food as a Factor*, 9.

40. T. C. Duncan, *How to Be Plump: Or Talks on Physiological Feeding* (Chicago: Duncan Brothers, 1878).

41. Harvey A. Levenstein, *Revolution at the Table: The Transformation of the American Diet* (New York: Oxford University Press, 1988), 12.

42. Food historian Jennifer Jensen Wallach recently reasserted the commonly held opinion that women during the late nineteenth century behaved properly by eating lightly and with an aura of disinterest, except when presented with sweets. See Jennifer Jensen Wallach, *How America Eats: A Social History of U.S. Food and Culture* (Lanham, MD: Rowman & Littlefield, 2013), 133; see also Laura Shapiro, *Perfection Salad: Women and Cooking at the Turn of the Century* (New York: Henry Holt, 1986), 72. This view needs to be revised in light of dietary records.

43. Jaffa, "Nutrition Investigations at the California Agricultural Experiment Station."

44. M. E. Jaffa, *Nutritional Investigations of Fruitarians and Chinese at the California Agricultural Experiment Station, 1899–1901*, U.S. Department of Agriculture Office of Experiment Stations Bulletin 107 (Washington, DC: U.S. Government Printing Office, 1901).

45. Ibid., 7.

46. Ibid.

47. Bean cheese normally refers to *fermented* tofu or, as it was more commonly called, "bean curd." Jaffa may have applied the "cheese" label by mistake to the unfermented product, a suspicion supported by the absence of regular tofu (or plain bean curd) from his published lists of foods.

48. The men ate, on average, approximately 4 ounces (118 g) of bread per man per day and just over half a pound (239 g) of yams per man per day.

49. The dentist's cook did not serve any cabbage. Members of his household favored a variety of other greens, including lettuce, mustard, and spinach.

50. Atwater, "American and European Dietaries."

51. Research locations included Montreal, Quebec City, Richmond, Rivière-du-Loup, Sherbrooke, Sorel, Saint-Hyacinthe, and St. John.

52. Atwater, "American and European Dietaries"; Atwater, *Methods and Results*.

53. W. O. Atwater and A. P. Bryant, *Dietary Studies in Chicago in 1895 and 1896*, U.S. Department of Agriculture Office of Experiment Stations Bulletin 55 (Washington, DC: U.S. Government Printing Office, 1898); Ellen H. Richards and Amelia Shapleigh, "Dietary Studies in Philadelphia and Chicago, 1892–93," in *Dietary Studies in Boston and Springfield, Mass., Philadelphia, Pa., and Chicago, Ill.*, ed. Lydia Southard and R. D. Milner, U.S. Department of Agriculture Office of Experiment Stations Bulletin 129 (Washington, DC: Government Printing Office, 1903).

54. Beef liver, bacon, chicken, and canned sardines also counted as secondary core foods. Other such items included macaroni, lettuce, string beans, rhubarb, canned corn, cucumbers, canned tomatoes, strawberries, raisins, and currants.

55. Carroll D. Wright, "Food Consumption: Quantities, Costs, and Nutrients of Food-Materials," in *The Seventeenth Annual Report of the Massachusetts Bureau of Statistics of Labor* (Boston: Wright and Potter, 1886), 307. The exact figure was 4.95 lb. (2.25 kg), but the Massachusetts Bureau of Statistics of Labor published food weights as purchased and made no allowances for waste. Here the bureau's quantities are reduced by 10 percent, the estimated average rate of food waste in American households at the time.

56. European immigrants represented in the early dietaries ate an average of 1.7 kg of foodstuffs per man per day. Native residents of Quebec took in 1.4 kg/m/d or approximately 3 lb.

57. For example, in Massachusetts the intake of animal-sourced protein averaged 54 g/m/d. This amounted to 13 g/m/d more than in Quebec.

58. The intake of fat generally in Massachusetts averaged 204 g/m/d; Quebec's residents averaged 109 g/m/d. The intake of animal fat in Quebec averaged 95 g/m/d; it averaged 195 g/m/d in Massachusetts.

59. C. D. Woods and F. R. Mansfield, *Studies of the Food of Maine Lumbermen*, U.S. Department of Agriculture Office of Experiment Stations Bulletin 149 (Washington, DC: U.S. Government Printing Office, 1904).

60. Joseph R. Conlin, "Did You Get Enough Pie? A Social History of Food in Logging Camps," *Journal of Forest History* 23, no. 4 (1979): 178–79.

61. Woods and Mansfield, *Studies of the Food of Maine Lumbermen*, 32.

62. Joseph Conlin assembled a list of fifty-one foods, which by 1900 were being served by lumber-camp cooks nationwide. See Conlin, "Did You Get Enough Pie?" 167.

63. J. V. G. A. Durnin and R. Passmore, *Energy, Work, and Leisure* (London: Heinemann, 1967), 71.

64. Woods and Mansfield, *Studies of the Food of Maine Lumbermen.*

65. Conlin, "Did You Get Enough Pie?" 182.

66. Robert E. Pike, *Tall Trees, Tough Men* (New York: W. W. Norton, 1967), 18.

67. Atwater and Bryant's *Dietary Studies of University Boat Crews* did not include Harvard and Yale's costs of provisioning. The cost here is an estimate based on information provided for college men at other schools where they were boarding as nonathletes. See Jordan, *Dietary Studies at the Maine State College*; Tower, "Dietary Studies at Western Reserve University."

Bibliography

Albala, Ken. "Culinary History." In *Routledge International Handbook of Food Studies*, edited by Ken Albala, 114–21. London and New York: Routledge, 2013.

Albright, J. A. "Pellagra in Tennessee." In *Pellagra*, edited by K. J. Carpenter, 58–61. Stroudsburg, PA: Hutchinson Ross, 1981.

Andrews, Sidney. *The South since the War: As Shown by Fourteen Weeks of Travel and Observation in Georgia and the Carolinas.* Boston: Tickner and Fields, 1866.

Atwater, W. O. "American and European Dietaries and Dietary Standards." In *Connecticut Storrs Station Report for 1891*, 106–61. Storrs, CT: Storrs School Agricultural Experiment Station, 1891.

———. "The Chemistry of Food and Nutrition." *Century Illustrated Monthly Magazine* 34, no. 1 (May 1887): 59–74.

———. "Foods and Beverages." *Century Illustrated Monthly Magazine* 36, no. 1 (May 1888): 135–40.

———. "How Food Nourishes the Body." *Century Illustrated Monthly Magazine* 34, no. 2 (June 1887): 237–52.

———. *Methods and Results of Investigations on the Chemistry and Economy of Food.* U.S. Department of Agriculture Office of Experiment Stations Bulletin 21. Washington, DC: U.S. Government Printing Office, 1895.

———. "Pecuniary Economy of Food." *Century Illustrated Monthly Magazine* 35, no. 3 (January 1888): 437–46.

———. "The Potential Energy of Food." *Century Illustrated Monthly Magazine* 34, no. 3 (July 1887): 397–405.

Atwater, W. O., and A. P. Bryant. *Dietary Studies in Chicago in 1895 and 1896.* U.S. Department of Agriculture Office of Experiment Stations Bulletin 55. Washington, DC: U.S. Government Printing Office, 1898.

———. *Dietary Studies of University Boat Crews.* U.S. Department of Agriculture Office of Experiment Stations Bulletin 75. Washington, DC: U.S. Government Printing Office, 1900.

———. "Studies of Dietaries." In *Connecticut Storrs Station Report for 1896*, 117–58. Storrs, CT: Storrs Agricultural Experiment Station, 1896.

———. "Studies of Dietaries." In *Connecticut Storrs Station Report for 1898*, 130–53. Storrs, CT: Storrs Agricultural Experiment Station, 1898.

Atwater, W. O., and C. D. Woods. *Dietary Studies in New York City in 1895 and 1896.* U.S. Department of Agriculture Office of Experiment Stations Bulletin 46. Washington, DC: U.S. Government Printing Office, 1898.

———. *Dietary Studies in New York City in 1896 and 1897.* U.S. Department of Agriculture Office of Experiment Stations Bulletin 116. Washington, DC: U.S. Department of Agriculture, Office of Experiment Stations, 1902.

———. *Dietary Studies with Reference to the Food of the Negro in Alabama in 1895 and 1896.* U.S. Department of Agriculture Office of Experiment Stations Bulletin 38. Washington, DC: U.S. Department of Agriculture, Office of Experiment Stations, 1897.

———. "Food Investigations and Publications." *Storrs Agricultural Experiment Station Bulletin* 15 (1895): 3–15.

———. "Studies of Dietaries." In *Connecticut Storrs Station Report for 1894*, 174–204. Storrs, CT: Storrs Agricultural Experiment Station, 1894.

———. "Studies of Dietaries." In *Connecticut Storrs Station Report for 1895*, 129–74. Storrs, CT: Storrs Agricultural Experiment Station, 1895.

Bane, Juliet Lita. *The Story of Isabel Bevier.* Peoria, IL: C. A. Bennett, 1955.

Bennett, John W., Harvey L. Smith, and Herbert Passin. "Food and Culture in Southern Illinois—a Preliminary Report." *American Sociological Review* 7 (1942): 645–60.

Bevier, Isabel. "Dietary Studies among the Negroes in 1898." In *Dietary Studies of Negroes in Eastern Virginia in 1897 and 1898*, by H. B. Frissell and Isabel Bevier, 27–45. U.S. Department of Agriculture Office of Experiment Stations Bulletin 71. Washington, DC: U.S. Government Printing Office, 1899.

———. *Nutrition Investigations in Pittsburgh, Pa., 1894–1896*. U.S. Department of Agriculture Office of Experiment Stations Bulletin 52. Washington, DC: U.S. Government Printing Office, 1898.

Bevier, Isabel, and E. C. Sprague. "Dietary Study at Lake Erie College, Painesville, Ohio." In *Nutritional Investigations at the University of Illinois, North Dakota Agricultural College, and Lake Erie College, Ohio, 1896 to 1900*, by H. S. Grindley, J. L. Sammis, E. F. Ladd, Isabel Bevier, and E. C. Sprague, 27–38. U.S. Department of Agriculture Office of Experiment Stations Bulletin 91. Washington, DC: U.S. Government Printing Office, 1900.

Bourke, John Gregory. *Compilation of Notes and Memoranda Bearing upon the Use of Human Ordure and Human Urine*. N.p.: Privately printed, 1888.

———. "The Folk Foods of the Rio Grande Valley and of Northern Mexico." *Journal of American Folklore* 8 (1895): 41–71.

———. "The Urine Dance of the Zuni Indians of New Mexico." In *Annual Meeting of the American Association for the Advancement of Science*. Ann Arbor, MI: Privately printed and distributed with the author's compliments, 1885.

Brillat-Savarin, Jean Anthelme. *The Physiology of Taste, or Meditations on Transcendental Gastronomy*. Translated by Arthur Machen. New York: Dover, 1960.

Burke, Cathryn Boyd, and Susan P. Raia. *Soul and Traditional Southern Food Practices, Customs, and Holidays*. Ethnic and Regional Food Practices. Chicago: American Dietetic Association; Alexandria, VA: American Diabetes Association, 1995.

Calhoun, Creighton Lee. *Old Southern Apples*. Blacksburg, VA: McDonald and Woodward, 1995.

Carpenter, K. J. "Editors Comments on Papers 31 through 37." In *Pellagra*, edited by K. J. Carpenter, 268–74. Stroudsburg, PA: Hutchinson Ross, 1981.

———. "The Life and Times of W. O. Atwater (1844–1907)." *Journal of Nutrition* 124 (1994): 1707S–14S.

Chambers, Robert, Richard Longhurst, and Arnold Pacey, eds. *Seasonal Dimensions to Rural Poverty*. Totowa, NJ: Allanheld, Osmun, 1981.

Chapin, Robert Coit. *The Standard of Living among Workingmen's Families in New York City*. New York: Charities Publication Committee, 1909. Reprinted, New York: Arno Press, 1971.

Conlin, Joseph R. "Did You Get Enough Pie? A Social History of Food in Logging Camps." *Journal of Forest History* 23, no. 4 (1979): 164–85.

Corson, Juliet. *Miss Corson's Practical American Cookery and Household Management*. New York: Dodd, Mead, and Co., 1885.

Cummings, Richard Osborn. *The American and His Food: A History of Food Habits in the United States*. Chicago: University of Chicago Press, 1940.

Cutler, Irving. "Jews." In *The Electronic Encyclopedia of Chicago*, edited by Janice L. Reiff, Ann Durkin Keating, and James R. Grossman. Chicago: Chicago Historical Society, 2005. http://www.encyclopedia.chicagohistory.org/pages/671.html.

Davidson, Allan. *The Oxford Companion to Food*. Oxford: Oxford University Press, 1999.

Dickins, Dorothy. *A Nutrition Investigation of Negro Tenants in the Yazoo Mississippi Delta*. Mississippi Agricultural Experiment Station Bulletin 254. Agricultural College: Mississippi Agricultural Experiment Station, 1928.

Digital and Multimedia Center, Michigan State University Libraries. *Dishes and Beverages of the Old South. Feeding America: The Historic American Cookbook Project*. Digital and Multimedia Center, Michigan State University Libraries. http://digital.lib.msu.edu/projects/cookbooks/html/books/book_66.cfm.

Diner, Hasia R. *Hungering for America: Italian, Irish, and Jewish Foodways in the Age of Migration*. Cambridge, MA: Harvard University Press, 2001.

Dirks, Robert T. "Diet and Nutrition in Poor and Minority Communities in the United States 100 Years Ago." *Annual Review of Nutrition* 23 (2003): 81–100.

———. "What Early Dietary Studies of African Americans Tell Us about Soul Foods." *Repast* 26, no. 2 (2010): 8–18.

Dirks, Robert T., and Nancy Duran. "African American Dietary Patterns at the Beginning of the 20th Century." *Journal of Nutrition* 131 (2001): 1881–89.

———. "Agriculture Experiment Station Studies and the History of Food Habits and Nutrition in the United States." *Nutritional Anthropology* 21 (1998): 6–8.

———. "Experiment Station Dietary Studies Prior to World War II: A Bibliography for the Study of Changing American Food Habits and Diet over Time." *Journal of Nutrition* 128 (1998): 1253–56.

Dirks, Robert T., and Gina Hunter. "The Anthropology of Food." In *Routledge International Handbook of Food Studies*, edited by Ken Albala, 3–13. London and New York: Routledge, 2013.

Drewnowski, Adam. "Obesity, Diets, and Social Inequalities." *Nutrition Reviews* 67, no. S1 (2009): S36–S39.

Drewnowski, Adam, and Barry M. Popkin. "The Nutrition Transition: New Trends in the Global Diet." *Nutrition Reviews* 55, no. 2 (1997): 31–43.

Du, S. F., B. Lu, F. Zhai, and B. M. Popkin. "A New Stage of the Nutrition Transition in China." *Public Health Nutrition* 5 (2002): 169–74.

Duncan, T. C. *How to Be Plump: Or Talks on Physiological Feeding*. Chicago: Duncan Brothers, 1878.

Durnin, J. V. G. A., and R. Passmore. *Energy, Work, and Leisure*. London: Heinemann, 1967.

Etheridge, Elizabeth W. "Pellagra." In *The Cambridge World History of Human Disease*, edited by Kenneth F. Kiple, 918–24. Cambridge: Cambridge University Press, 1993.

Farmer, Fannie Merritt. *Boston Cooking-School Cook Book*. Boston: Little, Brown, 1896.

———. *What to Have for Dinner, Containing Menus with the Recipes Necessary for Their Preparation*. New York: Dodge, 1905.

Fischer, Maureen M. *Nineteenth-Century Lumber Camp Cooking*. Exploring History through Simple Recipes. Mankato, MN: Capstone Press, 2001.

Floud, Roderick, Kenneth Wachter, and Annabel Gregory. *Height, Health, and History: Nutritional Status in the United Kingdom, 1750–1980*. Cambridge: Cambridge University Press, 1990.

Fogel, Robert W., Stanley L. Engerman, and James Trussell. "Exploring the Uses of Data on Height." *Social Science History* 6, no. 4 (1982): 401–21.

Forman, S. E. *Conditions of Living among the Poor*. Bulletin of the Bureau of Labor 64. Washington, DC: U.S. Government Printing Office, 1906.

Frissell, H. B. "Dietary Studies among the Negroes in 1897." In *Dietary Studies of Negroes in Eastern Virginia*, U.S. Department of Agriculture Office of Experiment Stations Bulletin 71, 7–25. Washington, DC: U.S. Government Printing Office, 1899.

Gabaccia, Donna R. *We Are What We Eat: Ethnic Food and the Making of Americans*. Cambridge, MA: Harvard University Press, 1998.

Gentile, Maria. *The Italian Cook Book: The Art of Eating Well, Practical Recipes of the Italian Cuisine, Pastries, Sweets, Frozen Delicacies, and Syrups*. New York: Italian Cook Book Co., 1919.

Gerrior, Shirley, Lisa Bente, and Hazel Hiza. *Nutrient Content of the U.S. Food Supply, 1909–2000*. Home Economics Research Report no. 56. Washington, DC: U.S. Department of Agriculture, Center of Nutrition Policy and Promotion, 2004.

Gibson, H. B., S. Calvert, and D. W. May. *Dietary Studies at the University of Missouri in 1895*. U.S. Department of Agriculture Office of Experiment Stations Bulletin 31. Washington, DC: U.S. Government Printing Office, 1896.

Gibson, H. B., C. D. Woods, and W. O. Atwater. "Studies of Dietaries." In *Connecticut Storrs Station Report for 1893*, 174–97. Storrs, CT: Storrs Agricultural Experiment Station, 1893.

Goel, M. S., E. P. McCarthy, R. S. Phillips, and C. C. Wee. "Obesity among US Immigrant Subgroups by Duration of Residence." *Journal of the American Medical Association* 292, no. 23 (2004): 2860–67.

Goldberger, J., G. A. Wheeler, E. Sydenstricker, and W. I. King. *A Study of Endemic Pellagra in Some Cotton-Mill Villages of South Carolina*. U.S. Public Health Service Hygienic Laboratory Bulletin 153. Washington, DC: U.S. Government Printing Office, 1929.

Goodyear, Caroline. "Household Budgets of the Poor: An Inquiry into the Dietary Standards and Habits of a Group of Tenement House Families in New York City." *Charities and the Commons* 16, no. 4 (1906): 191–97.

Goss, Arthur. *Dietary Studies in New Mexico in 1895*. U.S. Department of Agriculture Office of Experiment Stations Bulletin 40. Washington, DC: U.S. Government Printing Office, 1897.

——. *Nutrition Investigations in New Mexico in 1897*. U.S. Department of Agriculture Office of Experiment Stations Bulletin 54. Washington, DC: U.S. Government Printing Office, 1898.

Greenbaum, Florence Kreisler. *The International Jewish Cook Book: 1600 Recipes according to the Jewish Dietary Laws with the Rules for Kashering: The Favorite Recipes of America, Austria, Germany, Russia, France, Poland, Roumania, Etc., Etc.* New York: Bloch, 1919.

Grindley, H. S., and J. I. Sammis. "Dietary Studies at the University of Illinois." In *Nutritional Investigations at the University of Illinois, North Dakota Agricultural College, and Lake Erie College, Ohio, 1896 to 1900*, by H. S. Grindley, J. L. Sammis, E. F. Ladd, Isabel Bevier, and Elizabeth C. Sprague, 7–20. U.S. Department of Agriculture Office of Experiment Stations Bulletin 91. Washington, DC: U.S. Government Printing Office, 1900.

Haber, Barbara. "Culinary History vs. Food History." In *The Oxford Encyclopedia of Food and Drink in America*, edited by Andrew F. Smith, 301–3. Oxford and New York: Oxford University Press, 2004.

Haines, Michael R., and Richard H. Steckel. *Childhood Mortality and Nutritional Status as Indicators of Standard of Living: Evidence from World War I Recruits in the United States*. National Bureau of Economic Research Working Paper Series on Historical Factors in Long-Run Growth, Historical Paper 121. Cambridge, MA: National Bureau of Economic Research, 2000.

Hess, Alfred F., and Lester J. Unger. "The Diet of the Negro Mother in New York City." *Journal of the American Medical Association* 70, no. 13 (1918): 900–902.

Hilliard, Sam Bowers. *Hog Meat and Hoecake: Food Supply in the Old South, 1840–1860*. Carbondale: Southern Illinois University Press, 1972.

Hills, J. L. "Dietary Studies in Vermont Farmers' Families." In *Dietary Studies in Rural Regions in Vermont, Tennessee, and Georgia*, by J. L. Hills, Charles E. Wait, and H. C. White, 1–20. U.S. Department of Agriculture Office of Experiment Stations Bulletin 221. Washington, DC: U.S. Department of Agriculture, Office of Experiment Stations, 1909.

Hills, J. L., Charles E. Wait, and H. C. White. *Dietary Studies in Rural Regions in Vermont, Tennessee, and Georgia.* U.S. Department of Agriculture Office of Experiment Stations Bulletin 221. Washington, DC: U.S. Department of Agriculture, Office of Experiment Stations, 1909.

Hodgson, J. M., B. H. Hsu-Hage, and M. L. Wahlqvist. "Food Variety as a Quantitative Descriptor of Food Intake." *Ecology of Food and Nutrition* 32 (1994): 137–48.

Hooker, Richard J. *Food and Drink in America: A History.* Indianapolis, IN: Bobbs-Merrill, 1981.

Institute for Colored Youth at Cheyney. *Applied Domestic Science Daily Menus for the School Year and a Dietary Study for October.* Philadelphia: Press of E. A. Wright, 1909.

Institute of Medicine and National Academy of Sciences. *Dietary Reference Intakes for Energy, Carbohydrate, Fiber, Fat, Fatty Acids, Cholesterol, Protein, and Amino Acids: A Report of the Panel on Macronutrients, Subcommittees on Upper Reference Levels of Nutrients and Interpretation and Uses of Dietary Reference Intakes, and the Standing Committee on the Scientific Evaluation of Dietary Reference Intakes.* Washington, DC: National Academies Press, 2002.

Jaffa, M. E. *Nutrition Investigations at the California Agricultural Experiment Station, 1896–1898.* U.S. Department of Agriculture Office of Experiment Stations Bulletin 84. Washington, DC: U.S. Government Printing Office, 1900.

———. *Nutritional Investigations of Fruitarians and Chinese at the California Agricultural Experiment Station, 1899–1901.* U.S. Department of Agriculture Office of Experiment Stations Bulletin 107. Washington, DC: U.S. Government Printing Office, 1901.

Joint FAO/WHO/UNU Expert Consultation. *Energy and Protein Requirements.* World Health Organization Technical Report Series 724. Geneva: World Health Organization, 1985.

Jordan, W. *Dietary Studies at the Maine State College in 1895.* U.S. Department of Agriculture Office of Experiment Stations Bulletin 37. Washington, DC: U.S. Department of Agriculture, Office of Experiment Stations, 1897.

Kephart, Horace. *Our Southern Highlanders: A Narrative of Adventure in the Southern Appalachians and a Study of Life among the Mountaineers.* Knoxville: University of Tennessee Press, 1913.

Komlos, John. *Nutrition and Economic Development in the Eighteenth-Century Habsburg Monarchy: An Anthropometric History*. Princeton, NJ: Princeton University Press, 1989.

——. Preface to *Stature, Living Standards, and Economic Development*, edited by John Komlos, ix–xv. Chicago: University of Chicago Press, 1994.

Ladd, E. F. "Dietary Study of a Club of Women Students at North Dakota Agricultural College." In *Nutritional Investigations at the University of Illinois, North Dakota Agricultural College, and Lake Erie College, Ohio, 1896 to 1900*, by H. S. Grindley, J. L. Sammis, E. F. Ladd, Isabel Bevier, and Elizabeth C. Sprague, 21–26. U.S. Department of Agriculture Office of Experiment Stations Bulletin 91. Washington, DC: U.S. Government Printing Office, 1900.

Langworthy, C. F. "Food and Diet in the United States." *Yearbook of the United States Department of Agriculture*, 1908, 361–78.

Levenstein, Harvey A. "The American Response to Italian Food, 1880–1930." *Food and Foodways* 1, no. 1 (1985): 1–24.

——. *Revolution at the Table: The Transformation of the American Diet*. New York: Oxford University Press, 1988.

Longhurst, Richard, and Philip Payne. "Seasonal Aspects of Nutrition." In *Seasonal Dimensions to Rural Poverty*, edited by Robert Chambers, Richard Longhurst, and Arnold Pacey, 45–51. Totowa, NJ: Allanheld, Osmun, 1981.

Maclachlan, Emily Stevens. "The Diet Pattern of the South: A Study in Rural Sociology." Master's thesis, University of North Carolina, 1932.

Mahon, Brid. *Land of Milk and Honey: The Story of Traditional Irish Food and Drink*. Cork, Ireland: Mercier Press, 1998.

Mallinckrodt, E. *Dietary Studies with Harvard University Students*. U.S. Department of Agriculture Office of Experiment Stations Bulletin 152. Washington, DC: U.S. Government Printing Office, 1905.

Mayer, A. M. "Historical Changes in the Mineral Content of Fruits and Vegetables." *British Food Journal* 99 (1997): 207–11.

McCulloch-Williams, Martha. *Dishes and Beverages of the Old South*. New York: McBride Nast, 1913.

Messer, Ellen. "Season Hunger and Coping Strategies: An Anthropological Discussion." In *Coping with Seasonal Constraints*, edited by Rebecca Huss-Ashmore, John James Curry, and Robert K. Hitchcock, 131–41. Philadelphia: MASCA, University Museum, University of Pennsylvania, 1989.

Moore, Louise. "The Food of Women Living Away from Their Families." In *The Food of Working Women in Boston*, edited by Lucile Eaves, 65–100. Studies in Economic Relations of Women 10. Boston: Wright and Potter, 1917.

Murton, Brian. "Famine." In *The Cambridge World History of Food*, edited by Kenneth F. Kiple and Kriemhild Conee Ornelas, 1411–27. Cambridge: Cambridge University Press, 2000.

Page, Linda Garland, and Eliot Wigginton, eds. *The Foxfire Book of Appalachian Cookery*. New York: Gramercy Books, 1984.

Parloa, Maria. *Miss Parloa's Kitchen Companion: A Guide for All Who Would Be Good Housekeepers*. Boston: Estes and Lauriat, 1887.

———. *Miss Parloa's New Cookbook: A Guide to Marketing and Cooking*. New York: C. T. Dillingham, 1882. First published 1880 by Estes and Lauriat.

Paton, Diarmid Noël, J. Craufurd Dunlop, and E. Inglis. *A Study of the Diet of the Labouring Classes in Edinburgh: Carried Out under the Auspices of the Town Council of the City of Edinburgh*. Edinburgh: Otto Schulze, 1902.

Peterkin, Betty B. "Food Consumption Research: Parade of Survey Greats." *Journal of Nutrition* 124, no. S9 (September 1994): 1836S–42S.

Pike, Robert E. *Tall Trees, Tough Men*. New York: W. W. Norton, 1967.

Poe, Tracy N. "The Origins of Soul Food in Black Urban Identity: Chicago, 1915–1947." *American Studies International* 37, no. 1 (1999): 4–33.

Popkin, B. M. "The Nutrition Transition: An Overview of World Patterns of Change." *Nutrition Reviews* 62 (2004): S140–S43.

———. "The Nutrition Transition and Obesity in the Developing World." *Journal of Nutrition* 131 (2001): 871S–73S.

———. "The Nutrition Transition in Low-Income Countries: An Emerging Crisis." *Nutrition Reviews* 52 (1994): 285–98.

Popkin, B. M., and S. Du. "Dynamics of the Nutrition Transition toward the Animal Foods Sector in China and Its Implications: A Worried Perspective." *Journal of Nutrition* 133 (2003): 3898S–906S.

Rachman, Anne-Marie. *"Buckeye Cookery."* *Feeding America: The Historic American Cookbook Project.* Digital and Multimedia Center, Michigan State University Library. http://digital.lib.msu.edu/projects/cookbooks/html/books/book_33.cfm.

———. "Florence Kreisler Greenbaum." *Feeding America: The Historic American Cookbook Project.* Digital and Multimedia Center, Michigan State University Libraries. http://digital.lib.msu.edu/projects/cookbooks/html/authors/author _greenbaum.html.

———. *"The Italian Cookbook."* *Feeding America: The Historic American Cookbook Project.* Digital and Multimedia Center, Michigan State University Libraries. http://digital.lib.msu.edu/projects/cookbooks/html/books/book_71.cfm.

———. "Miss Parloa: Maria Parloa (September 25, 1843–August 21, 1909)." *Feeding America: The Historic American Cookbook Project.* Digital and Multimedia Center, Michigan State University Libraries. http://digital.lib.msu.edu/projects/cookbooks/ html/authors/author_parloa.html.

———. *"Mrs. Rorer's New Cook Book."* *Feeding America: The Historic American Cookbook Project.* Digital and Multimedia Center, Michigan State University Libraries. http://digital.lib.msu.edu/projects/cookbooks/html/books/book_54.cfm.

———. "Wilcox, Estelle Woods (1849–1943)." *Feeding America: The Historic American Cookbook Project.* Digital and Multimedia Center, Michigan State University Libraries. http://digital.lib.msu.edu/projects/cookbooks/html/authors/author _wilcox.html.

Richards, Ellen H., and Amelia Shapleigh. "Dietary Studies in Philadelphia and Chicago, 1892–93." In *Dietary Studies in Boston and Springfield, Mass., Philadelphia, Pa., and Chicago, Ill.*, edited by Lydia Southard and R. D. Milner, 37–98. U.S. Department of Agriculture Office of Experiment Stations Bulletin 129. Washington, DC: U.S. U.S. Government Printing Office, 1903.

Richards, Ellen H., and Marion Talbot. *Food as a Factor in Student Life.* Chicago: University of Chicago Press, 1894.

Rorer, Sarah Tyson Heston. *Mrs. Rorer's Every Day Menu Book: Giving a Menu for Every Meal in the Year; Menus for Weddings, Dinners, Receptions, and Many Other*

Social Functions; with Illustrations of Appropriate Decorated Tables. Philadelphia: Arnold and Company, 1905.

———. *Mrs. Rorer's New Cook Book: A Manual of Housekeeping*. Philadelphia: Arnold and Company, 1902.

Rosický, Marie. *Bohemian-American Cookbook: Tested and Practical Recipes for American and Bohemian Dishes (an English Language Translation of the Cook Book Published in the Bohemian Language and Compiled by Marie Rosický)*. 5th ed. Omaha, NE: Automatic Printing Company, 1949. First published 1915.

Rowntree, B. Seebohm. *Poverty: A Study of Town Life*. New York: Howard Fertig, 1902.

Scrimshaw, N. S. "Human Protein Requirements: A Brief Update." *Food and Nutrition Bulletin* 17, no. 3 (September 1996): 185–90.

Shapiro, Laura. *Perfection Salad: Women and Cooking at the Turn of the Century*. New York: Henry Holt, 1986.

Sinclair, Upton. *The Jungle*. New York: Jungle Publishing Company, 1906.

Singh, G. K., M. Siahpush, and M. D. Kogan. "Rising Social Inequalities in US Childhood Obesity, 2003–2007." *Annals of Epidemiology* 20, no. 1 (2010): 40–52.

Skelton, J. A., S. R. Cook, P. Auinger, J. D. Klein, and S. E. Barlow. "Prevalence and Trends of Severe Obesity among U.S. Children and Adolescents." *Academic Pediatrics* 9, no. 5 (2009): 322–29.

Sohn, Mark F. *Appalachian Home Cooking History, Culture, and Recipes*. Lexington: University of Kentucky Press, 2005.

Sombart, Werner. *Why Is There No Socialism in the United States?* White Plains, NY: M. E. Sharpe, 1976.

Stamm, Sara B. B., and the Lady Editors of *Yankee* Magazine, eds. Yankee *Magazine's Favorite New England Recipes*. Dublin, NH: Yankee, Inc., 1972.

Steckel, Richard H. "Heights and Health in the United States, 1710–1950." In *Stature, Living Standards, and Economic Development*, edited by John Komlos, 153–70. Chicago: University of Chicago Press, 1994.

———. "Slave Height Profiles from Coastwise Manifests." *Explorations in Economic History* 16 (1979): 363–80.

———. *Stature and Living Standards in the United States*. National Bureau of Economic Research Working Paper Series on Historical Factors in Long-Run Growth Working Paper 24. Cambridge, MA: National Bureau of Economic Research, 1991.

Steckel, Richard H., and Donald R. Haurin. "Health and Nutrition in the American Midwest: Evidence from the Height of Ohio National Guardsmen, 1850–1910." In *Stature, Living Standards, and Economic Development*, edited by John Komlos, 117–28. Chicago: University of Chicago Press, 1994.

Steinbock, R. T. "Rickets and Osteomalacia." In *The Cambridge World History of Human Disease*, edited by Kenneth F. Kiple, 978–80. Cambridge: Cambridge University Press, 1993.

Stitt, K. "Nutritive Value of Diets Today and Fifty Years Ago." *Journal of the American Dietetic Association* 36 (1960): 433–40.

Stone, Winthrop E. *Dietary Studies at Purdue University, Lafayette, Ind., in 1895*. U.S. Department of Agriculture Office of Experiment Stations Bulletin 32. Washington, DC: U.S. Department of Agriculture, Office of Experiment Stations, 1896.

Swan, P. B., and K. J. Carpenter. "Myer E. Jaffa: Pioneering Chemist in the Food and Nutrition Sciences." *Bulletin for the History of Chemistry* 21 (1998): 51–57.

Taylor, Joe G. *Eating, Drinking, and Visiting in the South*. Baton Rouge: Louisiana State University Press, 1982.

Tipton, Alice Stevens. *New Mexico Cookery*. Santa Fe: Bureau of Publicity of the State Land Office of the State of New Mexico, 1916.

Tower, O. F. "Dietary Studies at Western Reserve University." *Western Reserve University Bulletin*, n.s., 4 (1901): 146–64.

Valenze, Deborah. "The Culture History of Food." In *Routledge International Handbook of Food Studies*, edited by Ken Albala, 101–13. London and New York: Routledge, 2013.

Voorhees, Edward B. *Food and Nutrition Investigations in New Jersey in 1895 and 1896*. U.S. Department of Agriculture Office of Experiment Stations Bulletin 35. Washington, DC: U.S. Department of Agriculture, Office of Experiment Stations, 1896.

Wait, Charles E. *Dietary Studies at the University of Tennessee in 1895*. U.S. Department of Agriculture Office of Experiment Stations Bulletin 29. Washington, DC: U.S. Government Printing Office, 1896.

———. "Dietary Studies of Families Living in the Mountain Region of Eastern Tennessee." In *Dietary Studies in Rural Regions in Vermont, Tennessee, and Georgia*, by J. L. Hills, Charles E. Wait, and H. C. White, 21–116. U.S. Department of Agriculture Office of Experiment Stations Bulletin 221. Washington, DC: U.S. Government Printing Office, 1909.

———. *Nutritional Investigations at the University of Tennessee in 1896 and 1897*. U.S. Department of Agriculture Office of Experiment Stations Bulletin 53. Washington, DC: U.S. Government Printing Office, 1898.

Wallach, Jennifer Jensen. *How America Eats: A Social History of U.S. Food and Culture*. Lanham, MD: Rowman & Littlefield, 2013.

Washington, Booker T. *Up from Slavery: An Autobiography*. New York: Doubleday, 1901.

White, H. C. "Dietary Studies in Georgia." In *Dietary Studies in Rural Regions in Vermont, Tennessee, and Georgia*, by J. L. Hills, Charles E. Wait, and H. C. White, 117–36. U.S. Department of Agriculture Office of Experiment Stations Bulletin 221. Washington, DC: U.S. Government Printing Office, 1909.

Wigginton, Eliot, ed. *The Foxfire Book: Hog Dressing; Log Cabin Building; Mountain Crafts and Foods; Planting by the Signs; Snake Lore, Hunting Tales, Faith Healing; Moonshining; and Other Affairs of Plain Living*. Garden City, NY: Doubleday, 1972.

Wilcox, Estelle Woods. *Buckeye Cookery, and Practical Housekeeping: Compiled from Original Recipes*. Marysville, OH: Buckeye, 1877.

Woods, C. D. "A Study of Actual Dietaries." In *Connecticut Storrs Station Report for 1892*, 135–62. Storrs, CT: Storrs Agricultural Experiment Station, 1892.

———. "A Study of Dietaries." In *Connecticut Storrs Station Report*, 90–106. Storrs, CT: Storrs Agricultural Experiment Station, 1891.

Woods, C. D., and F. R. Mansfield. *Studies of the Food of Maine Lumbermen*. U.S. Department of Agriculture Office of Experiment Stations Bulletin 149. Washington, DC: U.S. Government Printing Office, 1904.

Wright, Carroll D. "Food Consumption: Quantities, Costs, and Nutrients of Food-Materials." In *The Seventeenth Annual Report of the Massachusetts Bureau of Statistics of Labor*, 239–328. Boston: Wright and Potter, 1886.

Zechenterd, Katarzyna. "Russians." In *The Electronic Encyclopedia of Chicago*, edited by Janice L. Reiff, Ann Durkin Keating, and James R. Grossman. Chicago: Chicago Historical Society, 2005. http://www.encyclopedia.chicagohistory.org/pages/1104.html.

Ziegelman, Jane. *97 Orchard Street: An Edible History of Five Immigrant Families in One New York Tenement*. New York: Smithsonian Books/HarperCollins, 2010.

Index

About the Author

Robert Dirks is emeritus professor of anthropology at Illinois State University. He has conducted research in areas of both food habits and nutrition worldwide. His publications include papers in the *Journal of the Royal Anthropological Institute, Current Anthropology, American Anthropologist, World Cultures, Journal of Nutrition,* and *Annual Review of Nutrition.* His book, *Come & Get It! McDonaldization and the Disappearance of Local Food from a Central Illinois Community,* traces a changing food culture from frontier days to the beginning of the twenty-first century.